Rejuvenation

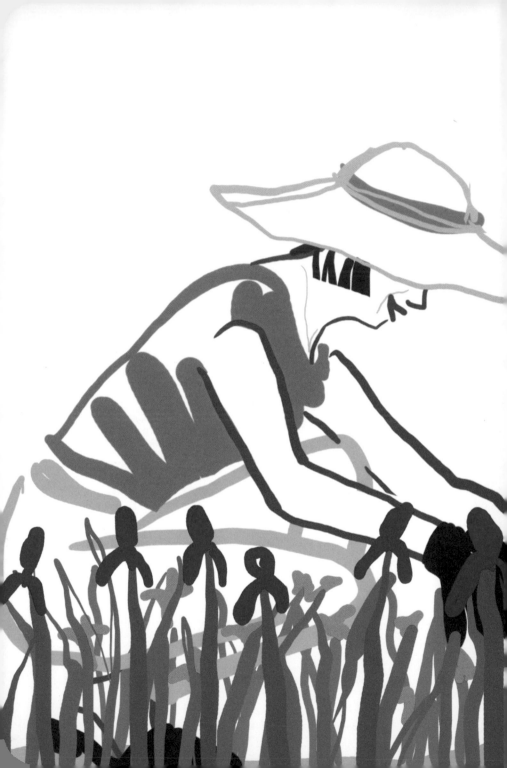

Rejuvenation

Spa Secrets for Menopause

BY MARY BETH JANSSEN
FOREWORD BY TONI BARK, M.D.
ILLUSTRATIONS BY AMY SAIDENS

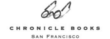

CHRONICLE BOOKS
SAN FRANCISCO

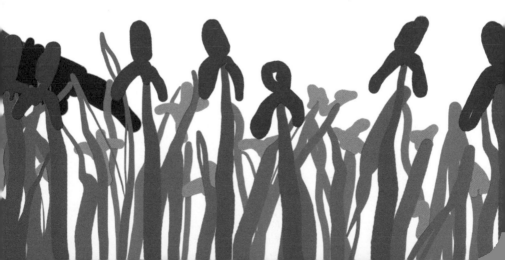

To the love and light of my life, James. And to my beloved parents, Nelly and Hubert. Mother, your example of acceptance and compassion knows no bounds.

Text copyright © 2007
by Mary Beth Janssen.
Illustrations copyright © 2007
by Amy Saidens.
Page 143 constitutes a continuation
of the copyright page.

Library of Congress Cataloging-in-Publication
Data available.

ISBN-10: 0-8118-5433-7
ISBN-13: 978-0-8118-5433-7

Manufactured in China.

Distributed in Canada by Raincoast Books
9050 Shaughnessy Street
Vancouver, British Columbia V6P 6E5

10 9 8 7 6 5 4 3 2 1
Chronicle Books LLC
680 Second Street
San Francisco, California 94107
www.chroniclebooks.com

Contents

FOREWORD BY TONI BARK, M.D.

It is an unusual woman who goes through menopause without complaint. In today's stressful and hyperkinetic world, we're often not tuned in to our body's rhythms, making it even harder to understand and cope with the effects of this physical, emotional, and spiritual change. So I say brava! for *Rejuvenation*. This book will help you attune to those rhythms and provide nurturing all-natural "therapies" for nearly every complaint I have heard from my patients to date.

We live in a time when drug companies rename old drugs in order to market them specifically to menopausal women, doctors push prescriptions for every complaint, and patients are confused and overwhelmed by conflicting information. Old antidepressants are renamed with new, feminine-sounding names, and anxialytics (derivatives of Valium) are repackaged as benign insomnia aids. Chalk is added to milk chocolate and sold as a healthful bone-building supplement!

While drugs may have their time and place in certain situations, they are not the "magic bullet" that so many physicians position them to be. Many American women go on prescription drugs for some aspect of their menopause when they could avoid doing so by learning how to more effectively manage stress as well as making some simple, positive changes in their lifestyle. Many prescription drugs can effectively treat a women's ailment, but they may also come with detrimental and long-term side effects.

A physician's oath is "First, do no harm," and with that in mind, I always opt for the most natural approaches to overcoming meno-pausal complaints—like those outlined in this book. For example, many menopausal patients come to see me after having been prescribed synthetic hormones by their previous physician. After running a profile of their hormones, I usually find that what they really need is a good resistance-exercise regime, a few dietary recommendations, and few, if any, hormones. In fact, my experience has shown that a large number of women can significantly control hot flashes with a shift in diet, an increase in physical activity, and the use of certain breathing techniques.

Although there is growing knowledge in the medical community about integrative approaches to menopausal symptoms, we still have a long way to go. See your health provider as needed, but know that you're the ultimate decision maker in your treatment—and that the mind/body therapies found in this book can serve as a healing, balancing adjunct to your physician's guidance. As Mary Beth has written in these pages, strive for an open and questioning relationship with your physician. Try to find a doctor who believes in a holistic approach, using the type of therapies featured here in tandem with traditional care. Be your own health-care advocate.

A smart woman will take charge of her health with as much knowledge as possible and find open-minded physicians who will work to understand her unique mental and physical makeup. And most of all, she'll use the vital information found in this book. Mary Beth has really done her homework and has useful advice for the treatment and prevention of the common ailments of menopause. Her recipes and practices are scientifically sound and exhibit a wide range of knowledge. From restorative yoga asanas to soothing massage techniques, Mary Beth Janssen has created a clear and concise practical guide to breezing through menopause. This is a most-needed reference, and exactly what my patients have been begging for!

INTRODUCTION

The "M" word has definitely come out of the closet. From menopause yoga classes and a hit Broadway musical to hot-flash cookbooks and night-sweat pajamas, menopause is fast becoming part of the pop culture landscape. It's even been the subject of a best-selling book. We have experienced *The Joy of Cooking* and *The Joy of Sex*, and now I propose the joy of menopause.

But first, Menopause 101: Menopause is not a disease, but a natural process where ovulation slows down, eventually coming to a halt, accompanied by a fluctuation and decline in reproductive hormones. It generally begins in our forties with a prelude called perimenopause, and culminates in our early fifties, when menses has stopped for at least twelve months. The one constant through it all is the shifting, swirling dance of our hormones. Depending on where we are on this journey, we may be experiencing less cool, calm, and collected versions of ourselves. If your mind has floated off into the ether, if your emotions have taken to swinging high and low, if your body is trying to put out fires or quench its thirst, the natural approaches, therapies, and "secrets" found in these pages will serve you well.

If we embrace menopause—instead of letting it scare the bejeezus out of us—this acceptance can rock our world! Menopause is not the end of womanhood, but, rather, a profound life passage that every woman will experience. The wise woman sees this time as an initiation into newfound values, exceptional creativity, and social consciousness. Now that we are beyond giving birth, we can focus on our own rebirth: a new assertiveness and commitment to protecting ourselves, our loved ones, and all of life. It's time to enjoy the wisdom that has grown within us over the years. This wisdom, effervescence, vitality, and humor—this soul—is our most powerful "secret" of all. This inner beauty is what captivates, hypnotizes, and turns heads when superficial beauty begins to fade.

Along with the spiritual manifestations of menopause, hormonal changes are causing physical changes in our body, as well as possible mental and emotional upheaval. It can be a little unsettling—or a lot unsettling—to experience puberty in reverse. But it can also be cathartic, mind-bending, and awe-inspiring. Trust that you'll get through this beautifully. Say to yourself, "I'm going to be fine." And keep on saying it. Because with the right attitude, you will!

This is our time to infuse our lives with rejuvenating practices that leave us feeling soothed and smoothed, energized and glowing, and balanced—inside and out. Because it is stress that precipitates many menopausal "sensations," we'll begin there, with centering and contemplative techniques for modulating stress and emotional upheaval. Next, we'll explore the changing landscape of our bodies—delving into a variety of therapies that will leave you feeling complete, capable, and sensual as you move from one phase of your life into another. And finally we'll consider matters of the heart, along with the essentials of bone and breast health in partnership with your health-care provider. All of this information combined can truly help you embrace your journey.

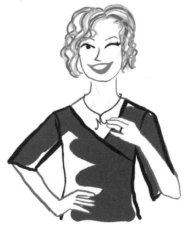

PART ONE

Mind over Menopause

The way we experience menopause is greatly connected to our lifestyle choices before, during, and after menopause. The good news is that from the moment you start integrating stress-management tech- niques, along with a delicious and nutritious diet, exercise, and carefully selected nutritional supplements, into your lifestyle, you can minimize if not eliminate menopausal sensations. That's huge! A posi- tive mental attitude will play a major role in this as well. If we view menopause as the end of our youth and sexuality, this period will be a more difficult one than if it is viewed as the next natu- ral phase of our life. Our outlook during this time can have a lot to do with the frequency and severity of any symptoms that we may experience.

Studies have proven how important the mind-body connection is to our well-being. As we think, so we become. Perhaps you've heard the saying: "Our issues are in our tissues." Unless we start each day with the powerful intention to nurture ourselves as much as pos- sible, self-defeating thoughts and activities can sabotage our goal to achieve wholeness and increase the probability of manifesting menopausal symptoms.

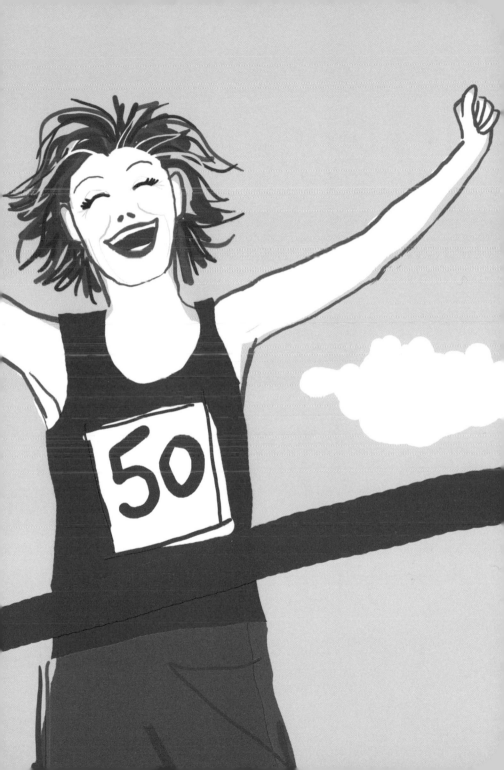

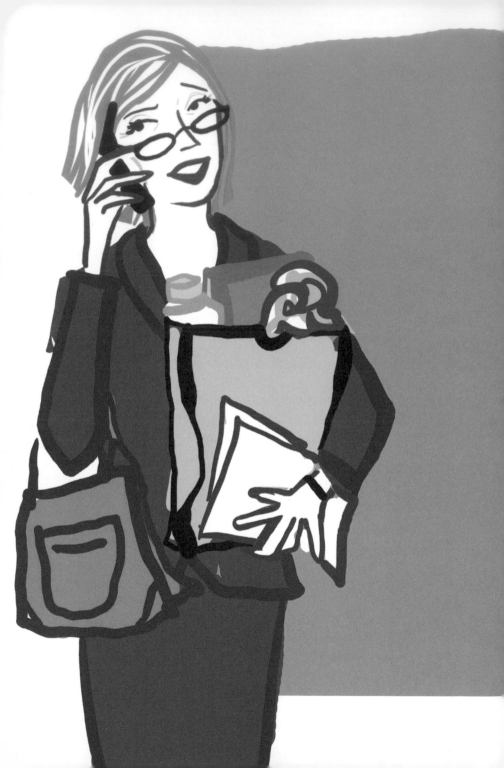

chapter 1

COPING WITH STRESS

S tress is at the root (make that root-squared!) of our hormonally challenged selves. It can throw off our body's natural balance of the five major hormones: estrogen, cortisol, testosterone, progesterone, and DHEA. It is irrefutable that uncontrolled emotional stress causes oxidative stress, or cellular aging. Science has proven that stress damages our DNA and can be the culprit behind wrinkles, gray hair, and those hot flashes—but also behind all forms of disease. And the shortening of our life span that results can be significant. What to do? One "prescription" is to put yourself at the top of your own to-do list. Get thee to the yoga mat, or meditate, or breathe deeply—and create a shift in your attitude. Emotional balance pays huge dividends for ourselves and everyone around us. You may need to look at your life and determine what needs to give. You may need to end a bad relationship, or switch jobs, or get rid of your cell phone, or get your finances organized, or take any number of other steps in order to take your life back.Ask yourself: Where can I let go of some attachments in order to live a simpler life? This kind of soul-searching can mightily deflect stress.

Most stress begins with our thoughts—that we don't have control over a situation, or the skills or resources to overcome it. If faced with a difficult situation, how we think about it may be as important, or more so, than the actual situation. (Studies have shown that those with the highest levels of *perceived* stress have greater cell aging.) So remember that *when a stressful situation occurs, we may not be able to control the situation, but we can control how we react to it.* Positive thoughts and healthy emotions, along with nurturing beliefs and practices, can dramatically shift stress responses in our body and lessen or stop the flow of detrimental stress hormones into our system—which ultimately can upset the entire hormonal apple cart!

By cultivating acceptance of this time in our lives, we're better able to face challenges that come our way. We become stronger and more resilient. Cultivate acceptance. Be kind to yourself. It can transform your life. And it can be unhealthy not to.

It's proven that women respond to stress differently than men. We may resort to what is called the "toxic triangle": unhealthful eating, heavy drinking, and self-criticism and despair. In order to cope with feeling tense, agitated, or out of control, we often end up doing damaging things to our bodies. Or we might worry excessively about what has happened, or what might happen, or dwell on how we should have done things differently. These responses interfere with our lives—our relationships, our work performance, and our overall well-being.

Unless we live in a Himalayan cave, stress is a fact of life. With the everyday demands life sends our way—the multitasking, the time compression that so many of us feel, the demands to achieve, and the constant exposure to misery and mayhem in the media—is there any wonder that so many of us are stressed? Our lives may include our own emotional baggage, relationship conflicts, financial pressures, work pressures, and simply feeling as if there is never enough time to accomplish what needs to get done. Many of us are caregivers for both our children and our aging parents—*and* we're also juggling a career, or facing retirement.

Other stressors include the environmental toxins we're exposed to through the food we eat, the air we breathe, and the water we drink—as well as the personal-care and household cleaning products that we use. Many chemicals are present in our surroundings—in clothing, building materials, carpeting, wallpaper, paint, and so on. Often they are not only carcinogenic but allergenic, and endocrine-disrupting in nature. We must try to lessen our exposure to as many of these toxins as possible. And today, more than ever before, healthful food, exercise, deep breathing, and nurturing thoughts are of tremendous benefit. It's essential to "detox" and rejuvenate our bodies in these ways so that our hormones can maintain some semblance of balance.

In our lives, we will all face traumas and tragedies—along with minor day-to-day stressors that can build to something major. This is why we strive to have a variety of healthful coping mechanisms to choose from. Following are some therapeutic approaches that will help you connect to your inner source of peace, enthusiasm, creativity, strength, and joy. Think of them as your toolbox and draw upon them whenever stress strikes.

MINDFULNESS

Mindfulness is the nonjudgmental awareness or "witnessing" of the moment and your place in it. Whether you're having a hot flash, eating a meal, washing dishes, brushing your teeth, making love, or dealing with the traffic jam you're in, try to be totally mindful of the experience. Stop resisting life, and let moments arise, as they are, without labeling them. When we're not mindful, life becomes less satisfying. We're always somewhere else, striving or longing for what's not there. But really, what's not there is you. When we're fully present, our life changes dramatically. We see the fullness of what *is*, and not what is lacking. Being fully present also gives you the knowledge to make choices about stressful situations (and if the problem can't be solved, then to learn how to better cope with it). You can fully embrace a moment because it nurtures you, or walk away from it because it will deplete you.

Mindfulness takes practice—but as with forming any new habit (which usually takes thirty days), it can become second nature. "Witness" your thoughts from the time you get up in the morning until you go to bed at night. Narrate your day to yourself. "Good morning, self . . . " Cultivate the habit of interrupting yourself to take note of what you habitually pay attention to and what you ignore. Choose a word, activity, or phrase to "trigger" your mindfulness if your awareness has lapsed—for instance, "be here now," or "pay attention." As you "witness" your thoughts, moods, activities, and sensations, you start to see what makes you feel good and not so good.

MEDITATION

Studies have shown that women who did 15 to 20 minutes a day of some form of meditative activity reported a 58 percent reduction in premenstrual symptoms and significantly reduced hot-flash intensity, and 90 percent were able to reduce or stop using sleep medications. These woman also displayed more positive attitudes toward their changing bodies—along with less anxiety and fewer negative thoughts.

Meditation refers to any practice where you deeply focus or reflect on something—like your breath, a prayer, a mantra (a chosen word such as love or peace), music, or a candle. Meditation elicits the "relaxation response," helping us connect with the core of our being. As thoughts come into our mind, we nonjudgmentally let them come and go like migrating birds, and gently come back to the object of our attention. This practice brings us to a deep inner silence where great healing and relaxation take place. We release tension in body and mind. We become calmer, clearer, more focused in our life, and more available to others. Meditation helps us let go of judgments—of ourselves and others—and helps us to put distance between events and our reactions. It teaches us to "not sweat the small stuff." And last but not least, it sparks our motivation to learn, grow, and stay curious about the world around us. It nurtures this sense of wonder, awe, and playfulness. Research has shown that meditation alleviates not only hot flashes, but also medical conditions ranging from hypertension to clinical depression to asthma. Meditation's tremendous rejuvenative powers become most profound when practiced every day.

MAKING THE CONNECTION WITH YOUR INNER SELF

Become as mindful as possible, witnessing everything that you do. Observe yourself reading this sentence right now. Be here now. When you shower, really feel the water on your skin. When you eat, really taste your food. When you crawl into bed tonight, observe yourself shifting from wakefulness to sleep.

✦   Commit to the power of breathing exercises, meditation, positive affirmations, creative visualization, and physical activities such as yoga, Pilates, tai chi, or ecstatic dance. Each practice serves to hone our sensitivity to mindfulness, allowing our spirit to soar into uncharted waters—and into the realm of infinite possibilities.

✦   Get lost in organic and sacred rituals. Burn a favorite candle or incense, then connect with the aroma, color, and movement of the flame. Play enchanting music, then hear each individual note as well as the harmony. Read your favorite poem or prayer aloud and listen to the rhyme and texture of the words.

- ✦ Walk in nature. Enjoy the sensual feast inherent in everything. See the smallest details in the trees, rocks and water. See the universe in a leaf. Feel the sun on your face, and the wind in your hair. Listen to nature's primordial sounds.

- ✦ Create a thing of beauty. Sketch, paint, mold clay, make a mosaic or an ornament.

- ✦ Construct an altar at home or at work. Make a special place for objects that have meaning for you—a loved one's photo, a rosary, or perhaps a quartz gem. Every time you see the altar, you are gently reminded of the spirit's presence, eliciting tranquility and centeredness.

- ✦ Let your soul be unleashed through writing. Keep a journal each and every day. Write down whatever is on your mind, without editing or censoring. You will experience many insights.

- ✦ Cultivate peace in a garden. This can involve an acre out back or a terra-cotta pot on your veranda. Visualize what your garden will look like after it receives loving care, and then set out to bring this beauty home. See your garden as a metaphor for your inner garden: a place for planting, weeding, and harvesting.

- ✦ Know that you are beauty personified. Spend a day on yourself, indulging in beautifying rituals. Visit a spa. Let a cadre of beauty professionals nurture you and treat you to an experience of sheer bliss. Or, give yourself a spa day at home.

- ✦ Tune in to the cosmic rhythms of the universe. Honor the sun, the moon, and the stars. Celebrate the seasons. Is it spring, with blossoms bursting open and a general resurgence of energy everywhere? See this as a metaphor for your mind-body physiology. Is it winter, when life returns deep into the earth for a season of introspection? Another great metaphor to feast on.

> ✦ Honor every significant stage in your life, as well as momentous stages in your loved ones' lives. This may mean something as seemingly small as cutting out one hour of television every night so that you can find quiet time to meditate, as well as honoring major life events such as giving birth, getting married, or losing a loved one. Honor them all!

VISUALIZATION

Visualization is a practice of forming positive images in the mind. It can be used for relaxation or to manifest desirable outcomes. Visualize a beautiful scene in a relaxing place. Become very intimate with every detail of this place. Use all your senses. Experience the colors, aromas, textures, and sounds. Feel the movement of the air. Remember to breathe deeply. Stay with this visualization for 5 to 10 minutes. Let your entire body relax into the scene. Once you get the hang of it, you will find this a very powerful technique for programming your subconscious to create desirable results, such as releasing fears, quelling stress, and achieving goals. Visualize loving relationships. Visualize experiencing joy. Visualize your body strong and toned. Visualize your skin smooth and glowing. You may just manifest what you visualize!

POSITIVE AFFIRMATIONS

A positive attitude is huge in managing stress. Optimism builds our resiliency to get over, through, and beyond challenges that come our way. It places us in solution mode instead of problem mode. Positive thinking enacts powerful effects on our mind and body. It raises energy levels and creates a can-do attitude. Studies show that positive affirmations raise the body's white blood cell count, giving a healthy boost to our immune system.

Positive affirmations help us become an optimist. With this practice we say a positive word, phrase, or sentence either silently to ourselves or out loud at any point where positive reinforcement is needed. One example could be "Every day, in every way, I'm getting better and better." Or "I'm proud of who I am." Another: "I'm cool, calm, and collected." Create your own positive affirmations that you can call on whenever your inner censor rears its ugly head with any form of negative self-talk.

COMPASSION

With so much stress around us, what can we do to bring peace and harmony into our lives? We can begin by having compassion for others—the ultimate sign of emotional maturity. I guarantee you that this practice will reward you richly. Compassion gives us understanding, patience, and empathy for ourselves and others. We become aware that we're all doing the best we can with the resources we have. When we try to understand that others may be acting out of pain, hurt pride, or low self-esteem, we become less judgmental, more tolerant, and more ready to forgive. And with a forgiving heart, we drop the burdens of anger, resentment, and sadness that contribute to our stress. When we learn how "to walk in someone else's shoes," we find it easier to open our heart and love unconditionally. Try this: As you move through your day, interact with people in a nonjudgmental and compassionate way. And remember that everyone is carrying some kind of burden. So be kind.

HEALING BREATH

If stress has gotten the upper hand, just breathe! It's one of the simplest yet most profound techniques for quelling stress. It helps you gain composure and some perspective in the face of troubling thoughts, moods, and emotions.

When done properly, breathing brings air into the lower portions of the lungs, where the oxygen exchange is most efficient. Our heart rate slows down, our blood pressure lowers, our digestion improves, our muscles relax, our anxiety eases, and our mind calms down. All bodily systems follow suit—including our hormonal system. Fresh, oxygenated blood energizes our brain, while the movement of lymph boosts immunity. It also releases those wonderful endorphins—our own natural mood-enhancing and pain-relieving chemicals. Anyone can use breathing to develop better sleep patterns, improve blood circulation, and increase mindfulness. Ah, sweet breath!

STRESSED? TRY BELLY BREATHING

Diaphragmatic breathing, also called "belly breathing," provides dramatic relief from stress (as well as hot flashes, night sweats, and so much more!). The diaphragm muscle is sandwiched between the lungs and abdomen. When we take a full, deep breath into the lungs, our diaphragm muscle presses down on the belly, moving it outward. When we exhale, the belly contracts inward. For many of you, this kind of breathing will feel counter intuitive (particularly in a culture where we're encouraged to "suck in our stomach," along with wearing tight belly-binding clothing!). But keep at it, and you'll get the knack of it.

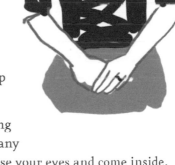

✦ Lie down—or sit comfortably, letting your hands rest in your lap. Let any tension in your body release. Close your eyes and come inside.

✦ Listen to and acknowledge your thoughts, feelings, and sensations in this present moment ("I feel hot," "I feel irritable," "I feel grateful," and so on.)

✦ Release any imbalance or negativity and send healing energy to yourself. Affirm positive thoughts. ("I am strong and in control." "I'm a beautiful and powerful woman.")

- ✦ Shift your attention to the gentle, rhythmic inflow and outflow of your breath.

- ✦ Inhale through the nostrils into the lowest part of the lungs and witness your belly moving outward. Do not raise your shoulders.

- ✦ Exhale and witness your belly moving inward. Make sure that you exhale completely before the next inhale.

- ✦ Without jerking or pausing in between the inhale and exhale, take 10 deep diaphragmatic breaths.

This kind of healing breath will have a cooling, calming, balancing effect on your bodily systems. Use it whenever you think of it, but especially when you feel any uncomfortable emotion or menopausal sensation coming on.

HEALING MOVEMENT

Physical activity is a blessing for our mind, body, and soul. It's simply vital to our well-being. Aside from antibiotics for a life-threatening infection, there's no medicine any doctor can prescribe that can affect our longevity and quality of life like regular exercise. It benefits all bodily systems, is a major stress-busting activity, improves sleep, boosts mood (those wonderful endorphins!), and helps in secreting excess hormones. It is also one of the most powerful beautifiers available to us. The more efficiently our nutrient-rich blood circulates, the more beautiful and healthy our skin, hair, nails, and eyes will be. Healing movement can be any form of physical activity. Try to include some cardiovascular, flexibility, and strengthening activity in your daily fitness regimen. Physical activity like yoga, Pilates, tai chi, and qigong encourages a balance between the mental and physical, as do long, delicious walks, dancing, gardening . . . and the like. These are all opportunities to slow down and be mindful of the moment.

NUTRITION

Nutrition is a major player in helping to deflect stress. In the midst of menopause, it has never been more important for us to eat in a hormone-friendly way. Eating a balanced diet of nutritious organic whole foods gives us tremendous energy, a strong, resilient body, and greater immunity to emotional as well as physical stressors. By selecting foods that fortify our arteries and veins, we are more able to absorb and use nutrients. Every cell in our body is working in physiological harmony, leading to glowing skin, lustrous hair, strong nails, and radiant eyes.

You may have heard the expression, "We are what we eat." Our nutritional intake has just this kind of power over all areas of our well-being. A whole-foods diet will go a long way toward modulating our hormonal balance and thus the sensations associated with menopause: hot flashes, a sluggish metabolism, weight gain, moodiness, and so much more. Diets high in refined sugar and starch cause insulin levels to spike, which can lead to an increase in estrogen as well as cortisol (a stress hormone) levels. Natural and organic foods that are certified free of hormones are very beneficial, especially at this time. (Commercially produced meat, eggs, and dairy products are full of synthetic hormones and antibiotics, which are often fed or injected into the animals to prevent disease or stimulate production.)

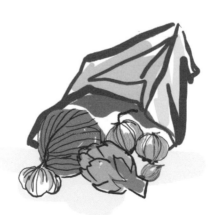

MASSAGE

Massage is a great way to release tension in the mind and body. Whether massaging our own skin or touching that of another, there's tremendous healing power in our hands. Visiting a massage therapist, enjoying a massage by the hands of a loved one, or treating yourself to a self-massage will make you feel cared for and touched on a sensory level that is incredibly beneficial. Massage releases a flood of natural feel-good chemicals into the bloodstream. It's been shown that the power of touch can reduce stress, increase levels of endorphins, ease pain, lift depression, and lower blood pressure. Massage is also an incredible beautifier for skin and hair, stimulating blood flow to the skin's surface. It increases the flow of blood and lymph throughout the entire body, aiding detoxification. A facial, massage, or body wrap can relieve tension, relax you, and clear your mind—all necessities, not luxuries, in the daily stresses of life.

Many middle-aged women have significant issues with bodily pain: arthritis, fibromyalgia, and so on. When under stress, the body tenses up. The fasciae—sleeves surrounding our muscle—tighten and bind the muscles into constricted positions. Stiffness and pain are felt in the fibrous tissues, usually deep within the muscles, though there's nothing wrong with the muscles themselves. Some believe that stiffness can also be the result of rigid thinking. Tension and fear result in the body gripping and cramping. All the more reason to meditate, do a daily self-massage, and occasionally visit a professional massage therapist.

AROMATHERAPY

Aromatherapy is the art and science of using essential oils (concentrated plant extracts) to relax, balance, and stimulate the body, mind, and spirit. These oils can boost confidence, help detoxify, soothe aching muscles, enhance metabolic and other bodily functions, and purify our environment.

You can use essential oils inhaled right from the bottle or placed on a cotton ball; you can also diffuse them (with a diffuser) into the air in your personal or work space, or add a few drops to massage oil or lotion and use for massage. Essential oils that are particularly helpful in treating menopausal symptoms include anise, bergamot, clary sage, coriander, fennel, geranium, jasmine, mint, and nutmeg. Certain oils are effective for relieving stress and enhancing mood; these include chamomile, lavender, and orange blossom.

HYDROTHERAPY

Since ancient times, bathing has been seen as a ritual that is synonymous with purifying, cleansing, and calming. Whether taking a shower, a bath, or enjoying a whirlpool—truly a nonprescription muscle relaxant—bathing is pure liquid tranquility. Water relaxes tight muscles, rejuvenates sore joints, and stimulates the release of endorphins, leaving you relaxed emotionally and physically.

The bath (and the shower as well) helps to nurture, balance, and release energy. Bathing washes away the pressures of daily life, while replenishing our well-being. Turn your bathtime into a relaxing, healing ritual by lighting a candle, playing music, and adding aromatic oils to the water (and dare I say a glass of organic Pinot Noir and an organic chocolate truffle, along with a juicy, spellbinding novel!). Or take an energizing shower, with alternating hot and cold water, to stimulate blood circulation and tone the skin. The water cure is always rejuvenative.

LAUGHTER THERAPY

It's easy to let a foul mood get the upper hand during menopause. Practicing lightheartedness can help. Did you know that children laugh on average four hundred times a day, adults only fifteen times? All the more reason to lighten up and have a good, side-splitting laugh as often as possible. Research shows that laughter really is good medicine. It releases endorphins into the bloodstream, improving mood. It also stops stress hormones and gives our immunity a powerful boost.

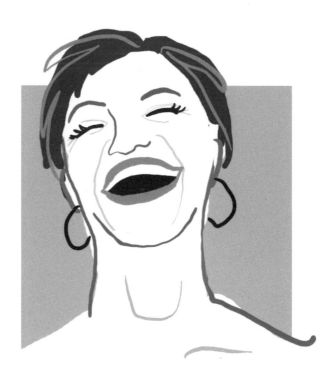

✦ Share the humor. When you hear or read something that tickles your funny bone, pass it on and laugh all over again.

✦ Choose your friends carefully. Those who make you laugh are a treasure. Distance yourself from those who are whiners or perpetually put out a doom-and-gloom vibe.

✦ Take up a new interest, preferably with someone you like. Rudimentary attempts at anything new can bring on hysterics, if you let it. Just remember, don't take yourself too seriously.

✦ Poke fun at yourself—or anything, for that matter. Look for the absurdities in daily life. There are so many of them.

✦ If you're not the naturally funny type, just concentrate on having fun! The laughs will come.

✦ Have some funny movies on hand, or make a point of renting them—and visit your library or one of the many hilarious Web sites that are devoted to all things humorous. Read their articles and their jokes, order a CD or a book.

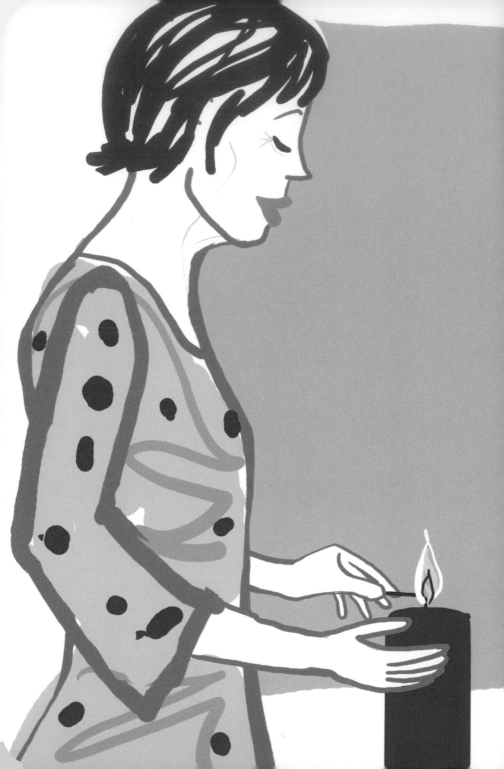

chapter 2

EMOTIONAL RESCUE

Hormonal fluctuations may cause mood swings and emotional upset. Yet other factors also contribute to changes in mood, including stress, insomnia, and life events that can occur in this stage of adulthood—such as the illness or death of a parent, grown children leaving home, and retirement (perhaps even forced retirement). Depression, anxiety, anger, and irritability can be seen as different forms of the same thing: holding on to emotional pain. Menopause is the perfect time to learn how to open up, accept life's twists and turns gracefully, and free yourself of emotional burdens. Acknowledge the feelings that you're having and don't simply "stuff" them. The repressed energy will keep circulating through your body's energy circuits. Emotional "cleansing" can be one of your best friends during this period of your life.

EMOTIONAL CLEANSING

We can really become a conditioned bundle of reflexes, wouldn't you agree? Letting your emotions control your life creates tremendous stress. And we already know how stress can affect us during menopause. Much of the stress we feel is relative to our perception of a given situation. When we learn to change our perceptions and attitudes toward stressful situations, we remove their ability to negatively affect us. This is a powerful step toward creating the harmonious balance that brings emotional well-being. This "emotional intelligence" begins with our taking responsibility for our feelings (after all, they're our feelings, no one else's).

To begin this cleansing process—adapted from one taught at the Chopra Center for Wellbeing—try observing your emotions. Begin simply, looking at one emotion either from your past or simmering in the present.

✦ Allow the feeling or "aura" of the emotion to well up. Emotions are thoughts connected to sensations in the body. That's why they're called "feelings."

✦ Identify the sensations you're feeling, such as frustration, bitterness, anger, shame, or sadness, as well as how they manifest in your mind and body: lightheadedness, stomachache, headache, backache, racing heart, and so on.

✦ Reflect on what the emotion reveals about you: a fearful ego, a need for approval, a need for control, a need for respect, a need for love. Be very clear on what it is that you feel you need but may not be getting.

✦ Verbalize or write down how the emotion makes you feel.

- Now, work on releasing the emotion and any painful body sensations. Affirm to yourself that you will do this. A ritual, such as ecstatic dance, singing, energetic breathing, or burning an aromatherapy candle or oils, can help to discharge the negative emotion.

- Celebrate the release. Take a luxurious bath. Go for a luscious walk through a park or forest preserve. Prepare and eat a nourishing meal. Listen to your favorite music. Get a massage.

- When you've finished the process, tune in to your mind and body. Do you notice a shift in attitude? Congratulations! You just gave yourself a tremendous gift. Use this process to dispel other unhealthy emotions. Give yourself a whole pile of gifts!

SOUL SEARCHING

On a daily basis, ask yourself: What do I want? Then write down what comes to mind, and look at this list every day. Edit your list as needed. Some suggestions:

- Physical/material—beauty, health, money, success, possessions.

- Emotional—loving relationships, respect, changes in attitude, the ability to get in touch with your true feelings, being centered or grounded, compassion.

- Spiritual—enlightenment, search for God or spirit, peace, laughter, harmony, joy, love.

And while you're writing in that diary, don't forget to write down the things that you're grateful for in your life.

TO FORGIVE IS DIVINE

Women tend to ruminate over things that others have done to them or things they've done that they regret. They go over them again and again, creating an energy-draining cycle. One of the ways out of this is to forgive ourselves or others. Toxic thoughts affect you and your well-being, not the person that you feel offended you. Holding on to being a victim keeps recycling negative energy. Lack of forgiveness prevents us from living in the present moment and experiencing joy. This affects our spiritual, mental, and physical wellness. Forgiveness has a tremendous healing effect. Let's be strong women and have a forgiving heart. Here are some steps to forgiveness:

✦ Consider a grievance or grudge against yourself or someone else. Go over the details without becoming emotionally charged. Deep breathing can help with this.

✦ Holding this image in mind, have the intention to forgive and release the grip it has on you. Say it out loud or to yourself: "I forgive myself [or_____] for the hurt, anger, bitterness that I [/they] caused."

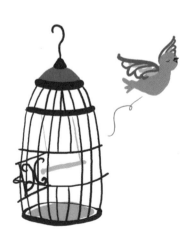

✦ Imagine how exhilarating it will feel when you take this load off your shoulders. Engelbert Humperdinck was spot-on when he sang, "please release me, let me go . . . " Very freeing indeed!

✦ Now, kiss and make up with yourself or someone that you've hurt, or who has hurt you. Ask for or offer forgiveness. Yes, it's daunting. But stand on your feet, and come from a place of inner strength.

+ Fortify your strength by asking for help from the depths of your soul, a higher power, nature, or your fellow humans.

+ Forgiveness engenders change and great healing. Please don't rush this. Bathe in it. You've created an energetic shift within yourself and your surrounding environment.

And remember, forgiveness does not mean that you condone what happened. But by forgiving, you release the constriction of energy surrounding the person or event. Instead of living in the past, you're joyfully living in the present.

GRIEVING: A PASSAGE TO TRANSFORMATION

The mid-life years can bring their share of difficulties—and sometimes deep sadness. It's important that we are able to navigate through these emotionally stressful times and appropriately mourn our losses. Loss comes in many forms (relationships, job, children leaving home, our "lost" youth), with the loss of a loved one the most profound. We are changed forever by loss, yet it may bring new depth of character, resiliency, and strength. Or, it may bring withdrawal, anger, and bitterness. We have a choice: we can accept and honor our pain, or we can deny it and keep it stored up inside us.

Grief is the all-encompassing and total response—mind, body, and soul—to the process of change. Change = loss = grief. Consider these "tasks" in grieving, whatever the loss:

+ Accept the reality of the loss.

+ Express the pain of the loss.

+ Nurture yourself emotionally, physically, and spiritually while experiencing the pain.

✦ Convert the lost relationship from one of presence to appropriate memory, using contemplative techniques such as mindfulness and visualization.

✦ Develop a new self-identity based on a life without your loss using some of the techniques in this book, including meditation, journaling, forging new relationships, and creating new experiences for yourself.

✦ Reinvest in your new reality.

✦ Relate your loss to the greater meaning of life.

✦ Stay connected to loved ones.

✦ Seek help if the pain is too great to work through alone.

There is no predictable or orderly progression to our experience of grieving. The goal in any loss is to work through it at your own pace. Also, tears can be beneficial—not a sign of weakness.

Often, true grief work begins after life has supposedly gone back to normal, your friends have stopped calling, and everyone thinks you should be "over it." Staying in touch with your inner voice and deeply caring for yourself can serve as the catalyst for deep healing. Acceptance and adjustment are born of this as well. The practices and therapies found throughout this book can renew your strength and optimism, and help you walk through the darkness into the light.

ACCEPTANCE

When we lose parts of ourselves once associated with our identity—beauty, youth, ambition—the pain can linger. This is where embracing the gifts of age can be freeing. Yoga's eight-limbed path to wholeness—including meditation, asanas (postures), and breath work—can be quite valuable in this process, because it takes us beyond the fact of our age. It turns us inward. As we explore our inner world and the strength and wisdom to be found there, we realize that we can rely on so much more than our looks. The happiness, peace of mind, and compassion that a yoga practice brings teach us not to fight what is, and to accept the process of aging. This doesn't mean that we stop looking after ourselves—or enjoying beautifying ourselves—whether coloring our hair, trying a new lipstick, or painting our toenails. It simply means we accept what is with grace, and stop grasping for that which is no longer there.

TRY THIS

Look in the mirror and take in every nuance of your face. See every line and crease. Spend some time studying your physical features. Now, close your eyes and "look" at who is inside doing the looking. Do you sense the spirit that is there? This is becoming the "witness." This exercise can help you in connecting with who you really are—instead of what you look like.

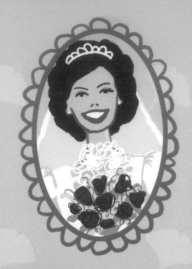
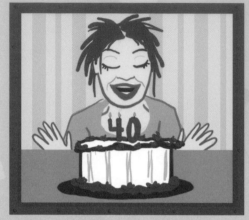
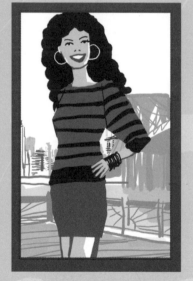
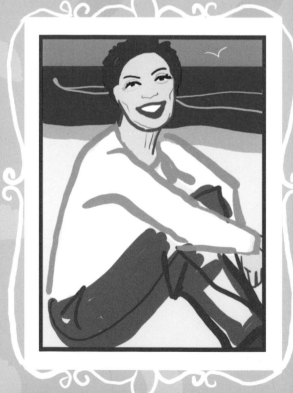

PART TWO

Our Changing Body

Hot flashes, an expanding waistline, wrinkled skin, thinning hair, sagging breasts (perhaps even sagging *everything*)—these changes and more may greet us at the onset of perimenopause. Some of us will experience just a smattering of these menopausal "sensations," while others will experience the *whole* enchilada. The difference is due to genetics as well as to our lifestyle choices leading up to menopause. Whatever the level of your body's changes, providing yourself with nurturing self-care will help you to navigate this passage and embrace the journey.

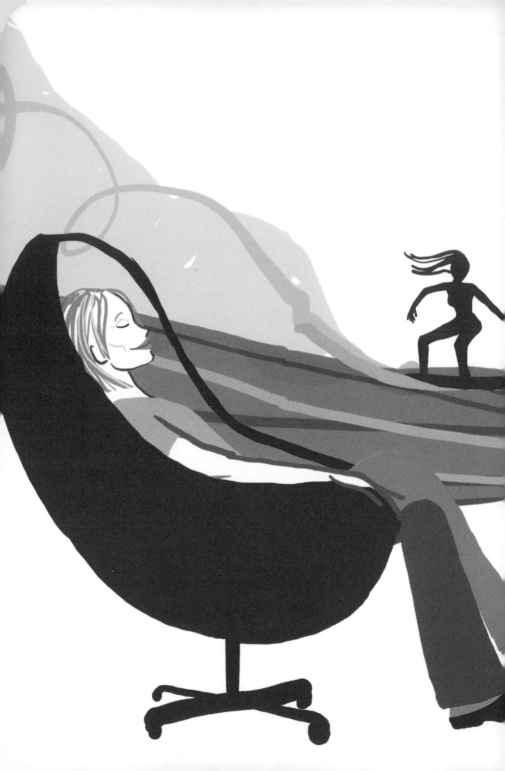

chapter 3

THE HOT FLASH, A.K.A. THE POWER SURGE

A natural yet potentially challenging sensation is the hot flash. More than 75 percent of American menopausal women will experience hot flashes—or what I like to call "power surges." Here are some ways to turn the power down a bit if you need to. ❧ Surges are thought to be caused by our body's thermostat located in the brain (the hypothalamus), as a result of hormonal imbalances and a compromised endorphin output (remember that endorphins help in elevating our mood and relieving pain). Unresolved stress can increase the amount and intensity of surges. These sudden rushes of hot energy begin in the chest, face, and neck and spread to other parts of the body. They can be subtle, or they can rage. Surges can last from 30 seconds to 5 minutes, and may happen a few times a year or as often as 30 to 40 times a day. They can also happen at any time of day or night (when they are called night sweats). ❧ What to do? In addition to consulting with your doctor, there are a number of natural ways to cool hot flashes and night sweats.

RIDE THE WAVE

Trying to control your hot flashes can make them more intense. Relax into it—instead of bracing yourself against it—and "ride the wave."

Sit down or lie comfortably, close your eyes, breathe deeply, and let the wave flow over you. Just ride that exhilarating wave in and onto solid ground—for those of you that like the surfing image. Visualization of this sort is very powerful. Create your own. Our body responds to the images that we create in our mind's eye. With visualization and deep healing breaths, you'll be pleasantly surprised at how your surges are lessened.

COOLING BREATH

Simply doing your belly breathing exercise (page 21) will provide hot-flash relief. However, this technique can step it up a notch, and is prized for its cooling and soothing qualities. If you're feeling heat or inflammation of any kind, this can help you quell the fire inside. And that includes any anger you may be feeling—an extra benefit here. As one friend shares, "I have learned to accept these flashes night and day and not become so angry, which adds to the intensity of the heat." Again, a matter of acceptance.

✦ Roll your tongue lengthwise to form a tube. The tip of the tongue will protrude slightly from the mouth.

✦ Inhale smoothly through your rolled tongue, making a hissing sound. (If the tongue will not roll lengthwise, curl the tip of the tongue back to touch the soft palate. With lips parted, inhale through closed teeth, making a hissing sound.) Follow the cool sensation down the throat and into the lungs.

- ✦ Relaxing your tongue and closing your mouth, exhale through your nostrils. The exhale will take a bit longer than the inhale.

- ✦ Repeat 5 to 10 times.

Practice this technique as often as desired, especially if you sense the onset of a surge. Release into your body, breathe, and Zen through it.

TAKING BATHS

Taking a bath at any time can be a healing ritual, especially if you're experiencing menopausal symptoms. Aroma adds a profoundly therapeutic element to the bath, and certain essential oils are especially helpful in reducing the number and severity of hot flashes.

Sage Advice

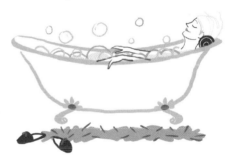

Sage and its relative, clary sage, are well known for their sweat-reducing and hot-flash-relieving properties. Epsom salts also provide amazing benefits: They help to draw toxins from the body, calm the nervous system, reduce swelling, and relax tight muscles. Epsom salts are also a natural emollient (serving to lock in moisture) and exfoliator for the skin. And both lavender and orange blossom are delightfully calming and cooling.

    1 cup Epsom salts

    10 drops clary sage essential oil

    3 to 5 drops lavender or orange blossom essential oil

Continued

Run a bath of body-temperature water. While the tub is filling, stir the Epsom salts into the water with your hand. When the bath is almost full, add the clary sage and lavender or orange blossom oils under the spout.

Now hop in and soak for 15 minutes. Gently towel dry. Then massage an organic body lotion over your entire body. Pure bliss, I say!

NOURISHING WISDOM

Phytoestrogens are a family of plant compounds that can mimic the action of estrogens in the human body. Increasing our intake of foods rich in phytoestrogens helps to reduce the frequency and severity of hot flashes.

Flavonoids are the dominant phytoestrogens in the human diet; so far, four thousand of them have been identified. They are divided into seven sub-families: flavones, isoflavones, flavanones, flavonols, coumestans, lignans, and chalcones. Isoflavones and lignans are currently considered to make the most significant contribution to the diet. Soy has become one of the more regularly "prescribed" phytoestrogens. If you're troubled by hot flashes, start working soy into your diet. Try cooked soybeans; snack on roasted soy nuts; throw tofu into soups, stews, pasta dishes, and stir-fries; pour soy milk on your cereal; use it in soups and puddings; or blend it into smoothies. Fermented soy foods like miso, natto, tempeh, and soy or tamari sauce are especially nutritious and easy to digest.

Widely varying foods from a whole-foods diet—fruits, vegetables, whole grains, and dried beans—will ensure that you're ingesting plenty of phytoestrogens every day. Some very common herbs and spices also have estrogenic properties, like licorice, nutmeg, oregano, thyme, and turmeric. When you shop, make sure that you're adding as many of these foods to your grocery cart as possible. Do remember that variety and moderation are important, because just as too much estrogen is unhealthy after menopause, too much phytoestrogen can also be of concern. So get your phytoestrogens from a widely varied whole-foods diet, rather than from one food, like soy, or from supplements. And remember to buy organic; don't expose yourself to toxic residues—including hormonal disrupting chemicals.

A Cautionary Note about Soy

Soy isoflavones create a form of hormonal or estrogenic activity that may stimulate estrogen-receptive diseases such as breast and ovarian cancer, especially in certain high-risk subgroups of women; researchers are currently investigating. So don't go overboard on the soy. Two to four servings a week should be fine. If in doubt, check with your doctor.

Berry Nice Smoothie

SERVES 1

Sooo refreshing—and sooo good for you too! The soy and flaxseed oil bestow their phytoestrogens to help reduce hot flashes, as do the bioflavonoids and vitamin C in the berries and juice. The yogurt and milk provide a healthy dose of your daily calcium requirement.

1 tablespoon high-lignan flaxseed oil

½ cup fresh or frozen strawberries, blueberries, or raspberries

½ cup fresh orange juice

½ cup plain low-fat dairy or soy yogurt

½ cup calcium-fortified soy milk or nonfat milk

1 small ripe banana

½ cup crushed ice or cracked ice cubes (optional)

In a blender, combine all the ingredients and blend until smooth. Pour into a large glass and slowly enjoy while affirming all the amazing benefits for your mind and body.

Limit or eliminate refined sugar, chocolate, alcohol, soda, coffee, and spicy foods, along with non-organic dairy products and red meat. They all promote menopausal sensations, especially hot flashes. They also elevate the level of acid in the blood, which contributes to a loss of calcium from our bones. If you choose to enjoy any of these items, make sure they are certified organic.

HERBAL THERAPY

Many herbal therapies are touted for their hot-flash-quelling abilities (among other benefits), and many have been used with very positive results. Chasteberry tree extract (also called vitex), dong quai, licorice, red clover, black and blue cohosh, sage, and white willow (also great for joint support and muscular aches and pains) are all very helpful. However, studies show that black cohosh is the premier herb to lessen or totally eradicate persistent hot flashes, night sweats, fatigue, mood swings (especially anxiety), inflammatory arthritis, and sleep disturbances. Take it in pill, tincture, or tea form. (In studies, 40 mg of a standardized extract was taken twice a day.) As with any supplements, it's important that they're high quality, and that you dose appropriately and consistently. Experts recommend trying black cohosh for two months to see if it works for you. Some well-known brands of herbal menopause remedies include black cohosh. Whichever form you use, consult your doctor and herbalist and follow their directions. Note: Many healing professionals advise using herbal therapies for the shortest period of time necessary to relieve symptoms.

BE A PHYSICAL ACTIVIST

Physical activity stretches us in every direction—physically, mentally, emotionally, and spiritually. Studies also show that it reduces the frequency and severity of hot flashes. In studies, women who exercised an average of 3½ hours per week on a regular basis passed through a natural menopause with no hot flashes whatsoever! That's only 30 minutes of physical activity every day.

TOTAL-AWARENESS WALKING

Be exquisitely present when walking! Wake up to the extraordinary beauty around you! And as you expose yourself to sun, sky, and wind, thank mother earth for all she does to nurture us. Witness your senses awakening—without the burden of thought or a running commentary going on in the mind. Keep your mind open and expansive. Your walk may be one where you're in a state of gratitude, with lots of positive self-talk. Or, concentrate on your body mechanics as

you walk: the swing of your arms, the way your feet hit the ground, the way your breathing feels as your pace changes. Visualize your body performing at its best—and how your vigorous walk balances your hormones, gives your heart a great workout, releases endorphins, and thoroughly energizes you.

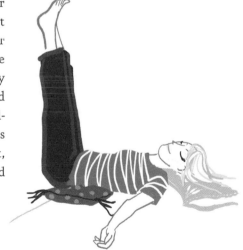

YOGA

Yoga postures soothe and calm the central nervous system, while helping to balance mind, body, and hormones. A consistent yoga practice can balance the endocrine system—the great hormonal regulator of the body—and relieve hot flashes and night sweats.

TURNING HOT FLASHES UPSIDE DOWN

Inverted yoga postures are valuable for their cooling and calming effects. Shoulder stands, headstands, legs-up-the-wall, forward bends, and Downward-Facing Dog are only a few of the many possibilities. Some believe that when we invert our bodies, we redirect the flow of prana—or life-force energy—inward toward the vital organs. Try inverting your body every day, and relish this posture's rejuvenative and balancing effect.

✦ Sit on the floor with one shoulder and hip next to the wall and your knees bent. Turn your legs upward along the wall until you are lying on your back. At first, you may not be able to place your buttocks flush against the wall. As you become more flexible, you will be able to bring them closer.

Optional: Have a folded blanket, pillow, or bolster close by to place under your buttocks, elevating your torso a bit higher. This further inverts your heart against the flow of gravity, reversing vascular flow and feeding fresh oxygenated blood to the brain.

✦ Bring your arms out by your sides—or form into a soft U shape with your hands facing above your head. Draw your shoulders down, away from your ears.

✦ Lengthen your neck along the floor, making certain your chin is lower than your forehead (place a folded towel under your head, if desired).

- ✦ Check in with your body and make certain there are no areas that feel strained.

- ✦ Breathe smoothly and evenly as long as desired.

- ✦ To come out of the pose, bend your knees to your chest and release toward the side onto the floor. Plant your hands on the floor to raise your body.

Mistified: A Cooling Body Mist

This cooling mist sends a message to the brain that says "Be cool—feel the tranquility." Many lovely sprays are available for purchase—however, I encourage you to make your own. The following recipe is about as pure and rejuvenative as you can get!

> 9 drops lemon essential oil (cleansing, uplifting, renewing)
>
> 7 drops peppermint essential oil (cooling, refreshing)
>
> 2 drops lavender essential oil (calming, relaxing, refreshing, toning, and cleansing)
>
> 8 ounces (1 cup) purified or filtered water

Combine the ingredients in a misting bottle. Use at intervals throughout the day, spraying your skin as well as the air around you. Spray your bedsheets—especially if you experience night sweats. Store for up to 1 week (but I'm certain you'll use it before then!). Shake before using.

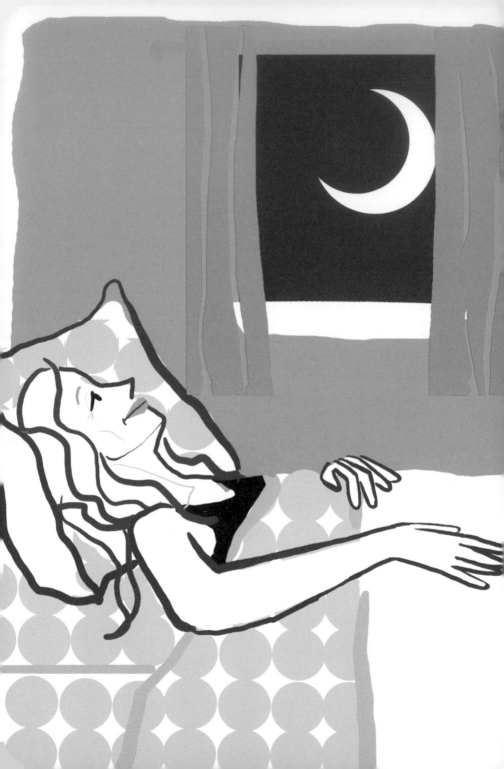

chapter 4

FATIGUE AND MEMORY LOSS

S tress, adrenal exhaustion, insomnia, night sweats—they can all bring on fatigue. Fatigue, in turn, is a major contributor to memory loss. This chapter offers a yin-and-yang approach to allaying fatigue, by sharing practices for increasing your energy during daylight hours while producing calming energy at night.

YOU DESERVE A BREAK TODAY

Fatigue means your circuits are overloaded. Giving yourself permission to be idle—and even a bit hedonistic—can recharge your batteries. Spend the day spinning your radio dial, watching clouds, and dancing to your own internal melody. Go for a walk with no destination in mind. Stare at the stars. Watch Swedish adult cinema, or spaghetti Westerns—one after another (whatever floats your boat, right?). If you can't take the whole day off, at least schedule little breaks through the day: afternoon tea, a lunch with friends, a nap, meditation, time to write in your journal. Every little bit helps.

REJUVENATIVE YOGA

Aches and pains, shifting moods, and mind-numbing fatigue may have to do with the health of our adrenal glands. If the adrenals are exhausted because of habitual stress, they are unable to increase their hormonal output to compensate for the lower output of our ovaries due to menopause. Poses that bend the lower back, such as the Bridge, the Cobra, and the Bow, tonify the kidneys, nourish the adrenal glands, stimulate the liver, and alleviate fatigue. The Bridge pose is a beginning back bend that anyone can enjoy and add to her daily practice.

✦ Lie on a yoga mat with your knees bent and your feet hip width apart and close to your buttocks. Your arms are by your sides.

✦ Relax and begin to watch the gentle in-flow and out-flow of your breath. As you let your body sink into the mat, feel your back lengthen and release.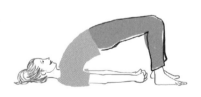

✦ Firm your buttocks and gently draw your tailbone toward your heels to protect your lower back. Pressing your feet into the floor, slowly lift your spine upward toward the sky as you inhale—thrusting your pelvis as high as is comfortable.

+ Keep breathing smoothly. Feel your back, glutes, and thigh muscles strengthening. You may stay in this pose for a few breaths or longer if desired.

Optional: While in the posture, you may join your hands on the floor underneath your back to further open the heart center and stretch through the shoulders.

+ As you exhale, slowly roll back down to the earth. Feel each vertebra touch down until finally the sacrum area of the spine touches the mat.

STIMULATING BREATH

This breathing pattern is great anytime you're feeling lethargic, fatigued, or depressed. It sends oxygenated blood circulating through the body and dispels carbon dioxide. It also stimulates the abdominals and digestive organs, massages the spinal column, and increases the circulation of lubricating fluids. If you're feeling a bit sluggish, this one will do the trick. Use it often.

+ Sit comfortably, with your spine straight and your eyes closed.

+ Place both of your hands on your abdomen.

+ Inhale slowly and passively. The belly moves outward.

+ Vigorously and forcefully exhale through the nose, while drawing the stomach tightly inward.

+ Repeat this passive inhalation and forceful exhalation 10 times.

+ Once comfortable with this technique, you can use it for up to 60 seconds.

Note: This technique should not be used if you have untreated heart disease.

GET YOUR Z'S

If your hormones are fluctuating, it can be challenging to get 7 to 8 hours of uninterrupted sleep. Estrogen stimulates the central nervous system, while progesterone has a relaxing effect. So, if we're churning out too much estrogen (as is common in perimenopause) and there's not enough progesterone to keep the estrogen in check, sleeplessness and anxiety may result. During the night we are in full detox mode, shedding the physical, mental, and emotional challenges of the day. Sleep deprivation zaps mental and physical energy and disrupts hormone levels, heart rate, blood pressure, and body temperature. It also wreaks havoc with serotonin levels, which affect our sense of well-being. If insomnia, night sweats, or mind chatter prevents you from drifting off or you awaken and can't drift back to sleep, consider the following:

THE WIND-DOWN ROUTINE

Develop a nightly routine for going to bed. Try to go to bed and get up at the same time every night and morning. Regular sleep hours help your nervous system learn when to turn on and off. And if you simply can't fall asleep, get up and do some quiet activity until you're overcome by sleepiness. Here are some other ways to encourage sound sleep:

✦ Meditate each day to release stress and clear your mind.

✦ Exercise for at least 30 minutes each day. Regular exercise can decrease the time it takes to fall asleep and increase total sleep time.

✦ Sip a cup of chamomile tea or warm milk with honey about an hour before bedtime and feel the relaxation seep through your body and mind. Note: Do not use chamomile every night, and avoid completely if you are allergic to ragweed.

- ✦ Valerian supports the nervous system and helps with persistent insomnia. Try using it in combination with other nerve-calming herbs like lemon balm, skullcap, oat straw, lady's mantle, and lavender, in tea, capsule, or tincture form. Also consider kava kava, passion flower, and hops—all very calming and anxiety relieving. You can also add these herbs to bath water, in tea or tincture form, to improve sleep.

- ✦ Take a warm bath before bed. Tie ½ cup rolled oats in a cheese-cloth square and add a few drops of lavender essential oil. Add this to your bath as the tub is filling with warm water. Use the bag as a washcloth to smooth the soothing, slippery oats over your body.

- ✦ Consider 5-HTP (5-hydroxytryptophan). It improves sleep, diminishes hunger, and is mood-uplifting. It boosts serotonin levels, which strongly influence sleep, appetite, and mood. It can also be very beneficial in managing bodily aches and pains—whether fibromyalgia or other musculoskeletal ills. Try 50 to 100 mg of 5-HTP, three times a day.

- ✦ Use a diffuser or light a natural aromatherapy candle in your bedroom. (Before drifting off, blow out the candle, please!) My favorites for relaxation are rose, lavender, ylang-ylang, geranium, and clary sage.

- ✦ Read inspiring material or listen to relaxation CDs or melodic music that effortlessly lulls you to sleep.

✦ Keep your bedroom dark and cool. Darkness signals the pineal gland to release melatonin, which not only makes us sleepy, but also stimulates the immune system, regulates estrogen, and may even lower our risk of heart attack and cancer. Sweet dreams!

✦ Do not have a large meal within three hours of bedtime, though a small protein snack—such as a few almonds or a small amount of low-fat yogurt—before bed may help promote a restful sleep by helping your body maintain normal blood sugar levels throughout the night. Avoid sugary or starchy snacks before bed, as they can lower blood sugar levels during the night. Avoid hidden sources of caffeine such as chocolate, green tea, soft drinks, and some herbs like yerba maté.

✦ Don't drink wine just before bed. Alcohol not only raises estrogen levels but also stimulates the central nervous system, so it may make you feel drowsy at first, but then rebounds to disrupt sleep. Excessive alcohol also throws into disarray our master internal clock that synchronizes all body systems, including hormone production, immune function, and sleep.

✦ Avoid vigorous activity in the hours just before bedtime. (Other than lovemaking, of course!)

TWO-TO-ONE BREATHING

This breathing pattern stimulates the parasympathetic nervous system—that part of our nervous system responsible for slowing down the heartbeat, lowering blood pressure, and creating harmonious brain-wave patterns.

✦ Consciously slow down your exhalation so that it is twice as long as your inhalation: For instance, try counting to 3 on your inhale, then to 6 on your exhale.

✦ Contract your abdominals to help in increasing the exhalation.

+ Focus on making each breath as smooth and even as possible, without any pauses or shakiness.

+ If you are having trouble going to sleep, lie on your back and take 8 breaths, then turn on your right side and take 16 breaths, then turn on your left side and take 32 breaths. Chances are you won't finish this exercise before drifting off to la-la land.

KEEP YOUR MENTAL EDGE

Forgetfulness and the inability to concentrate are commonly associated with menopause. Fatigue can be one of the culprits—zapping not only energy, but brain function. While some memory loss may be the result of estrogen decline, it may also be due to insufficient oxygen and nutrient supply to the brain. Though the brain weighs only 3 pounds, it utilizes about 20 percent of the oxygen supply of the entire body! Any therapy that enhances the function and flexibility of the blood vessels and the supply of blood, oxygen, and nutrition to the brain will be very beneficial. Consider these natural brain boosters:

+ Get enough sleep. It's proven that a lack of sleep trashes our memory and learning abilities.

+ Don't worry, be happy. Stress in all its forms creates tremendous aging of body and mind, including the portion of our brain responsible for memory retention. In studies, chronic worriers were 2.4 times more likely to develop Alzheimer's than those not prone to worry. Meditate, use positive affirmations, get a massage—but do whatever it takes to allay your anxiety and fears.

✦ Reach out to others. Those with a strong network of family and friends show less mental decline than those without familial ties when given cognitive tests over a twelve-year period.

✦ Regular exercise dramatically boosts oxygen to the brain. It's a major stress buster and mood enhancer. A major study showed that women who were physically active in their fifties and early sixties had the best memories in their seventies and beyond. And all it took was just ninety minutes a week to make a difference!

✦ Exercise your brain. Brain challenges keep your cognitive skills sharp. Watch game shows, play cards or chess, do crossword puzzles or brainteasers, learn a new language or how to play an instrument. Learning something new creates neural connections in the brain that help to stave off age-related memory loss.

✦ Eat Mediterranean. This diet is linked with lower rates of age-related cognitive decline. It features lots of fruits and vegetables, whole grains, potatoes, beans, nuts, and seeds. Olive oil is at the center of this diet. It includes plenty of fish, while dairy products, eggs, and poultry are consumed in low-to-moderate amounts. Little red meat is eaten. Wine is consumed in low-to-moderate amounts (it contains antiaging polyphenols).

✦ Drink moderately. Older women who enjoy one glass of wine, beer, or a cocktail each day scored higher on memory and other cognitive tests than both teetotalers and heavy drinkers.

✦ Do consider the herb ginkgo biloba. Its circulation-increasing benefits are especially helpful for forgetfulness (as well as relieving cold hands and feet). It increases blood flow to the brain and enhances energy production in that organ, improving the transmission of nerve signals, which are so important to memory.

✦ Research shows that writing things down helps to reinforce what we want stored in our brains. Use a notebook, or buy one of those fancy journals. And the more you do it, the more organized and less forgetful you become.

Stinging-Nettle Tea: An Infusion of Pure Energy Makes 1 cup

Long appreciated for its medicinal uses, stinging nettle is chock-full of vitamins and minerals, and is an amazing energy tonic. It's an excellent source of vitamins A, D, E, and K—as well as bone-building calcium, magnesium, potassium, boron, silicon, and zinc. It also has detoxifying properties, and can strengthen the adrenal glands, therefore making it a powerful therapy for fatigue. Make friends with stinging nettle, and along with added vim and vigor, you'll encourage a healthy heart, flexible bones, beautiful skin, and thicker hair.

1 teaspoon dried nettle, or 2 teaspoons minced fresh nettle leaf

1 cup boiling water

Honey to taste

Place the nettle in a tea strainer in a cup and add the boiling water. Cover the cup with a lid and infuse for up to 10 minutes before removing the herbs. Add honey and drink warm, or let cool and pour over ice.

Make in quantity in order to enjoy several cups over the course of the day; Use at least 1½ teaspoons (20 g) dried nettle leaf or 2 teaspoons (30 g) fresh per 2 cups of water. Place the nettle in a pot or jar and fill with boiling water. Cover and brew for up to 1 hour. Strain and drink hot or iced.

Ginseng to the Rescue

Siberian ginseng is a very specific herbal tonic for the adrenals. It helps with stress and fatigue.

Mix 3 parts Siberian ginseng root with ½ part cinnamon stick pieces and ½ part licorice root. Infuse, following the recipe outlined above. For something a bit different, cover in brandy and steep for 2 to 3 weeks. Sip like a cordial.

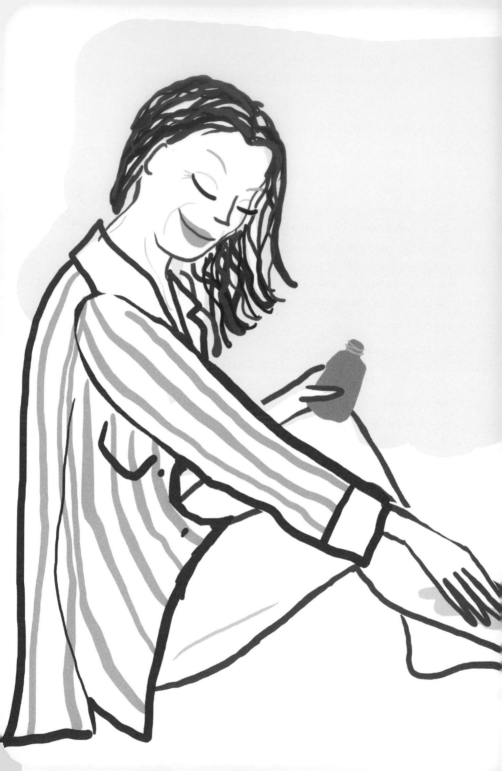

chapter 5

OUR CHANGING APPEARANCE

A change in metabolic function, digestion, or BMI (Body Mass Index) can alter the female body in many ways, including weight gain and "shape-shifting"—where formerly toned areas begin to jiggle and sag—along with gastrointestinal upset/bloating, cold hands and feet, and breast changes such as tenderness and loss of firmness. And, let's not forget: dry everything, including mucous membranes, skin, hair, and eyes. ¶ Check with your doctor to eliminate the possibility of hypothyroidism, which is common in menopausal women. Many symptoms (fatigue, intolerance to cold, weight gain, hair loss, dry skin, depression) ascribed to menopause may instead be due to low thyroid functioning.

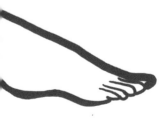

ALTERED STATES

Are your clothes fitting a bit too snugly for comfort? Many of us find that our body composition shifts as we age. Our body starts to lose muscle mass, and fat increases. (Especially if we are inactive.) Our weight may stay the same, but our waist has gotten bigger. Gravity also comes into play, no matter how active we are. You might also notice fat shifting into the abdominal area. Having conferred with your physician that nothing is amiss, consider the following:

OPTIMIZE YOUR DIGESTION

There is no doubt that as we age, our metabolism starts to slow down, and with it our ability to efficiently digest, absorb, and eliminate the food that we eat. Certain techniques can stoke the flame, enhancing our digestive and metabolic processes.

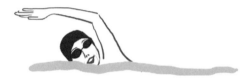

+ Shake up your exercise routine. Your body may have adapted to your new metabolism. Keep adding new and varied activities so your body is challenged to respond by trying to maintain a healthy body composition. Now is the time to add strength training to your routine. After age thirty, everyone starts losing muscle mass. Because muscle is so metabolically active, less muscle means we need fewer calories. Nothing will beef up muscles and calorie burning like weight training.

+ At the same time, you will need to step up your cardio activities. Kick up the frequency, intensity, and time allocated to your routine. For instance, if you're walking, increase your intensity level (walk faster) and/or increase your distance (walk farther). Consider wearing a weight vest as you walk. Remember that you don't want to be doing the same thing day after day, week after week. Consider seeing a personal trainer.

+ If you're exercising 30 minutes at least 5 days a week and your middle won't budge, you may be genetically predisposed to store more fat here. We can't change the body shape we inherited, but we can reduce overall body fat and tone the middle with exercise. If you're doing all this, and your belly is still flabby or your weight won't budge, then make sure that you're working at the right intensity for fat loss—at least 60 to 85 percent of your target heart rate (220, minus your age). Also, do core-strengthening exercises such as Pilates, or cardio that has core-toning benefits, like rowing, kickboxing, and swimming.

+ Review your nutritional intake. Our diet, weight, digestion, and metabolism are intimately connected. Diet can be the culprit in a slow and steady weight gain that creeps up on us. There isn't any one-size-fits-all metabolism fix. However, with a slow-down in metabolism, our nutritional needs may change. What has worked so comfortably up until now may no longer be appropriate.

THE INTUITIVE VERSUS STRESS EATER

Become an intuitive eater. Eat delicious, high-quality food—but slowly, in moderation, and with great pleasure. Don't get caught up in a diet mentality. This only creates stress, because we feel we're depriving ourselves. More stress equals more of the stress hormone cortisol circulating through our blood, while depositing fat in our belly area—among other places. How so? When we are stressed out, cortisol sends us searching for ice cream or other high-calorie foods to replenish the energy our body believes it spent in handling the stressful event. If chronically stressed, your body keeps churning out cortisol, causing you to continually reach for sugary, starchy, and fat-laden foods. This makes your blood sugar levels rise dramatically, then come crashing down (along with the resultant fatigue). Insulin is released into the bloodstream to handle the blood sugar, and over time this can create insulin resistance, a precursor to diabetes.

(Consider having a lipid density profile, since dense LDLs are a sign of insulin resistance.) Since the energy from this food intake is not spent on an activity, the fat deposits itself in the belly area. It's a vicious cycle, but one that we can control, as we learn coping techniques for managing stress—including healthful eating.

✦ Make whole, unprocessed foods like whole-grain bread and fresh vegetables the mainstay of your diet (they contain fiber and nutrients that keep blood sugar levels stable).

✦ Get the right balance of proteins, fats, and carbs with every meal or snack. High- and refined-carb diets rapidly raise, then lower, blood sugar, wreaking havoc with insulin levels. Protein and fat in our diet help slow down the absorption of carbs, keeping blood sugar levels steady. If we don't get enough protein, fat, and fiber, our body cranks out even more cortisol. This also triggers cravings.

✦ Don't skip meals. This can leave you ravenous and reaching for sugary/high-carb foods. Experts claim that grazing throughout the day on healthful foods is the best way to keep the metabolism humming along at its optimal best.

✦ Physical activity in all its forms not only brightens our mood but reduces cortisol and improves our overall stress resilience. Weight training not only provides cortisol control but also revs up our metabolism, helping us to tone and slim down at the same time.

So get a handle on the stress, ladies. Create pockets of peace through-out your day. Sidestep stress whenever you can and avoid situations that push your buttons.

Last but not least, supplement wisely with antistress nutrients.

✦ Magnesium and the B vitamins are well known for their relax-ation and mood-lifting benefits. Take 400 mg of magnesium and at least 100 percent of the recommended daily allowance of the B vitamins every day. If, after a couple of weeks, you find you need a further boost in managing stress, try adding the herb holy basil.

✦ Holy basil reduces cortisol and helps our body adapt to stress. Experts recommend 400 mg two times a day. Also called tulsi, it comes in tea form as well.

✦ If there's a stressful event on the horizon, try L-theanine. It's an amino acid in green tea that controls cortisol and helps you to relax within 30 minutes of ingesting, without any side effects. You can take 50 to 150 mg to keep you calm. Check with your doctor if you're on any prescription medicines. Experts say that L-theanine can be taken indefinitely.

THE FIBER CONNECTION

Fiber is a boon for weight control. It is not broken down by the body, so it cleans out residue in the digestive tract as it works its way through the body, thus aiding in digestion. A fiber-rich diet also reduces the risk of digestive diseases from diverticulitis to colon can-cer, and may reduce blood cholesterol levels. United States dietary guidelines advise that adults consume 25 to 30 g of fiber a day. Good sources of dietary fiber include cereals, nuts, whole grains, fruits, and vegetables. In a pinch, you can use supplements like psyllium husks to boost your daily fiber intake.

✦ Ginger tea promotes rapid and complete digestion, and increases intestinal tone and peristalsis (the movement of the bowels). It is also an excellent anti-inflammatory and detoxifier. To make it, bring water to a boil in a non-aluminum saucepan, add grated fresh ginger, and simmer for 2 minutes. Pour into a cup and add lemon juice and honey to taste. Make a thermos of this tea to sip through the day.

✦ Sipping warm water (with a bit of lemon) throughout the day will hydrate and cleanse bodily tissues. It keeps the metabolism moving along as well.

✦ One or two tablespoons of aloe vera juice taken twice a day will improve digestion and aid elimination.

✦ A shake or two of bitters in a glass of mineral water after eating has a marvelous effect on the digestion. It also alleviates the feeling of bloatedness.

NOURISHING WISDOM: A MINDFULNESS APPROACH

So many of us gobble down our food, rarely stopping to truly taste and appreciate it. Since it takes a full twenty minutes for our brain to register fullness, if we eat too quickly we will end up eating more than our body needs. This severely compromises the way we digest and metabolize food. Many of us could use a gentle reminder to be mindful when eating. Digestion begins in the mouth with the release of saliva and the thorough chewing of our food. If we eat with full awareness and appreciation, we'll automatically eat less and enjoy more. We'll hear our body saying, "I'm *sooo* satisfied. Perhaps I don't need that second helping after all!"

AN EATING MEDITATION

Be fully present while eating. Don't just feed your taste buds. Let food nourish all your senses. The more engaged you are with the smell, textures, colors, even the sounds of your food, the more deeply it will satisfy you and the less likely you'll overindulge. To learn the fine art of eating with spirit, try this eating meditation:

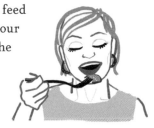

+ Settle yourself into a comfortable place with your food—whether you're eating a meal or a snack. Minimize distractions. No TV!

+ Give thanks to every person and circumstance that brought you this food—the farmer who lovingly planted the seed, the sun's life-giving energy that helped it grow, and so on. This includes whoever prepared the food, including yourself.

+ Look closely at the food. Become intimate with its shape, form, and texture. Use all your senses. Take in the colors. Touch the food. Smell the aromas. Let the food rest for a moment on your lips. Can you feel the saliva beginning to flow in your mouth? You should! All these sensory steps enact the digestive process.

+ After putting a morsel of food in your mouth, chew thoroughly, tasting the explosion of flavors. Notice how your jaw, tongue, and the muscles in your face move as you chew.

+ When you swallow, mentally follow the food down your esophagus and into the stomach. Pay attention to any stomach sensations. Maintain this level of mindfulness throughout your meal.

+ Do not gulp down beverages—especially cold drinks—during this eating meditation (or any meal!). It hampers digestion.

+ As you continue relishing each bite, you will begin to feel the sensation of fullness.

- ✦ After finishing your meal, sit for a few moments. Breathe evenly and naturally. Give thanks for this food and its life-giving sustenance.

- ✦ After a few reflective moments, get up and go for a brief walk—5 to 10 minutes will do. This will enhance the digestive process.

Now, think back over the entire process. Did you feel as if you were in super-slow motion? That's great! This is how we are meant to take in nourishment. If you did nothing else other than follow this practice with your entire food intake, you would not only maintain or lose weight, but you would transform the entire eating experience into one of joyful celebration.

MASSAGE YOUR BELLY

Regularity rules! Irregular bowel function and abdominal distress can go hand-in-hand. If you have an upset stomach or feel bloated, try rubbing your belly. There's lots of lymphatic tissue (which moves toxins out of the body) in this area. It feels so good, and it's very effective. Since the belly is the site of the 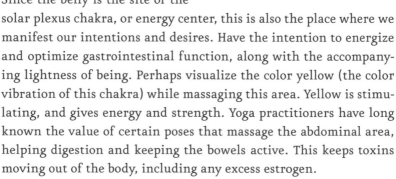 solar plexus chakra, or energy center, this is also the place where we manifest our intentions and desires. Have the intention to energize and optimize gastrointestinal function, along with the accompanying lightness of being. Perhaps visualize the color yellow (the color vibration of this chakra) while massaging this area. Yellow is stimulating, and gives energy and strength. Yoga practitioners have long known the value of certain poses that massage the abdominal area, helping digestion and keeping the bowels active. This keeps toxins moving out of the body, including any excess estrogen.

Stomach Massage Oil

These essential oils are stimulating, purifying, and vitalizing for the abdominal area as well as the entire nervous system.

> 1 ounce plant oil, such as sweet almond oil, coconut oil, olive oil
>
> 2 to 3 drops rosemary essential oil
>
> 2 to 3 drops peppermint essential oil
>
> 2 to 3 drops lemon essential oil

Mix the plant oil and essential oils. Work between the palms, then place both hands on your belly, fingers pointing toward each other, and begin to rotate the hands clockwise over the entire abdominal area. Visualize the energy from the oils and the massage strengthening your digestive processes and healing whatever ails you. Do this for as long as you like. It's so soothing!

Yoga Stomach Massage: You can also try a yoga approach: Sitting comfortably, place your balled fists on either side of your abdomen just below the navel. Now bend forward, with your torso folding over your balled fists. Hold for several deep belly breaths before straightening up. Work up to a minute or longer. This compression is a "wake-up" call for your intestines.

BREAST ESSENTIALS

Fat cells can make breast size and shape vary. Whether before, during, or after menopause, loss of fat cells and/or inadequate support can create sagging, droopy breasts. The breasts have no muscle tissue to hold them up. You want perky? Then build those pectorals and the muscles around the perimeter of the chest. These are the muscles that, when well toned, provide the supportive underpinnings for ample busts, while providing a boost for smaller busts. If you can add swimming to your routine, all the better—use the aptly named breaststroke to enhance your bustline.

These chest exercises will build the muscles surrounding the breasts, making them appear lifted and fuller. If you don't already have them, invest in a set of hand weights. Begin with the lightest-weight ones. These exercises can serve as inspiration for starting a free-weight routine to tone and benefit the entire body.

THE DUMBBELL INCLINE CHEST PRESS

+ Lie on your back on an incline bench, step aerobic bench, ottoman, or coffee table. Keep your lower back in a flat or neutral position.

+ Hold a dumbbell in each hand at the sides of your torso at chest level.

+ While exhaling, raise the dumbbells to a straight-arm position (elbows not locked).

+ Hold the dumbbells directly over the upper chest. The ends of the dumbbells should be in contact with each other, with your palms facing forward.

+ Inhale as you lower the dumbbells until they are at either side of your chest.

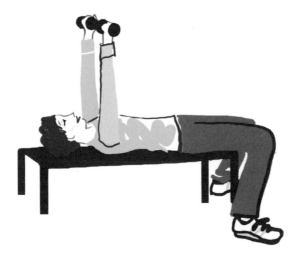

THE DUMBBELL INCLINE CHEST FLY

✦ Lie on your back on an incline bench, step aerobic bench, ottoman, or coffee table. Keep your back in a neutral position.

✦ With a dumbbell in each hand, extend your arms straight out to
   the sides, parallel to the floor. Keep your elbows slightly bent.

✦ On the exhale, lift your arms over your chest toward each other
   until the weights are almost touching. This movement actually seems like a large hugging motion.

✦ While inhaling, return to the starting position.

Do 10 to 12 repetitions of each exercise on three alternate days of the
week. You can work up to three sets of 10 to 12 reps. Make sure to
lower the weights in between each set and counter-stretch to release
held tension.

THE (LAZY WOMAN'S) DO-ANYWHERE PECTORAL LIFT

This isometric exercise can be done anywhere, anytime, to strengthen
the pectorals. No equipment is needed.

✦ Reach your arms out in front of you. Now, bend your elbows and
   grasp your forearms on either side just below the elbow.

✦ Breathe in through your nostrils, then breathe out and tighten
   your grip, pressing your forearms into your hands on either
   side. You will feel the contraction in your chest. Hold for a
   count of 5. Repeat 10 times.

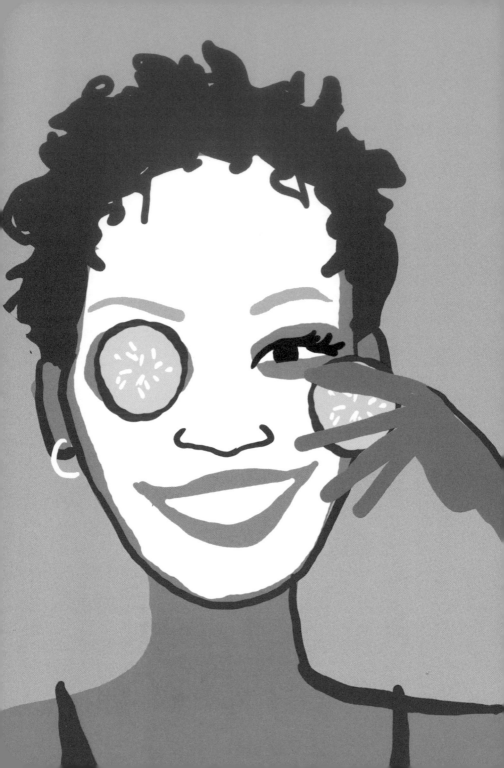

chapter 6

OUR CHANGING SKIN

Estrogen is a hormone that in the right amount maintains the moisture content of skin cells, along with the skin's strength, elasticity, and tone. As our hormonal balance begins to shift, our skin may dramatically change. A decrease in estrogen and oil production leads to thinner, more sensitized skin. Lifestyle choices and skin treatment, along with a change in the way our skin produces collagen and elastin (the skin's vital connective tissue), can create dry, lackluster skin, wrinkles, loss of skin tone, and various skin conditions like acne and rosacea. Here are some natural approaches to maintaining moist, toned, and glowing skin.

PROTECTING THE SKIN BARRIER

As we go through menopause, the epidermal layer of our skin doesn't slough off as easily and the skin doesn't retain as much moisture as it once did. The skin's support fibers, collagen and elastin (in the inner dermal layer), also start to break down and thin over time, and our skin becomes less pliable. The trick is to encourage the regular turnover of skin cells while maintaining the skin's natural acid mantle, the combination of sebum and perspiration that the body secretes to moisturize the skin's surface. This can help in maintaining or repairing collagen and elastin in order to preserve the skin's strength, elasticity, and resiliency.

THE HOLISTIC APPROACH TO RADIANT, DEWY SKIN

Healthy skin is alive with vibrating energy. It's radiant, smooth, supple, elastic, and moist. It also has a slight flush to it from optimal blood circulation. This kind of skin shows that lymph fluid is removing toxins and boosting immunity. Stress is under control, antioxidants are preventing free-radical damage, and hormones are balanced. The oil and sweat glands are bathing the skin with just the right amount of natural oil and moisture, which in turn maintains the skin's natural acid mantle. All the while, the skin is experiencing a constant state of renewal, turning over and shedding skin cells in a sort of healthful internal dance.

Here are a few perfectly natural ways to beautiful skin.

+ Reduce stress. Stress hormones rob our skin of its nourishing blood supply, create free radicals, and depress the immune system, disturbing the skin's balance and appearance. As you learn to relax, your skin cells will follow suit. Happy thoughts create happy cells in the body. Visualize beautiful skin. Meditate, breathe deeply, dance, or do whatever it takes to relax and reinvigorate yourself, calming your hormones *and* your skin.

+ Eat right. A varied diet with a balance of proteins, complex carbohydrates, good fats, and plenty of natural antioxidants provides all the daily requirements to generate healthy skin. High-quality protein helps skin growth and regeneration. Eat fruits and vegetables in abundance, along with whole grains, legumes, nuts, a bit of poultry and fish (particularly those rich in omega-3s, like salmon), and no or low-fat dairy. Every day, take a high-quality multivitamin with antioxidants, and omega-3s in the form of fish oil or flaxseed—along with at least two 500-mg capsules of borage or evening primrose oil. Your skin and hair will benefit immensely. Eliminate foods that spike blood sugar and insulin levels, especially anything made from white flour and white sugar, both inflammatory for the skin. You can also do your skin a world of good by reducing saturated animal fats and avoiding artificial ingredients and chemical pollutants. Alcohol, caffeine, and spicy foods can decrease barrier function and increase skin reactivity and inflammation.

✦ Sun protection. Although limited sun "baths" (early morning or late afternoon for 15 to 20 minutes) can be valuable for our body's metabolization of vitamin D, sun exposure is the number-one cause of premature skin aging and wrinkles. One of the best ways to protect the skin is to wear a moisturizing sunscreen with SPF 15 or higher. Choose one that blocks both UVA and UVB rays and contains titanium and zinc as active ingredients. Wear it anytime you're exposed to sunlight—whether outdoors or indoors (through windows).

✦ Stop smoking. Not only has it been proven that smoking initiates an earlier menopause, but it also exacerbates a wide variety of menopausal symptoms. Smoking is a major cause of massive skin damage, severely compromising the skin's ability to repair and rejuvenate itself. Create a powerful visualization around releasing this habit for good. Go see a therapist or a hypnotist, get the patch—do whatever it takes to stop smoking. Remember that one puff of a cigarette creates over a billion free radicals in your body. Very toxic indeed!

✦ Bathe in moisture. Water is the cheapest and most effective skin moisturizer, bar none, so drink up. It's absolutely essential for proper hydration, keeping the skin moist and plumped, supple, soft, and clear. It improves the skin's barrier function and helps the skin resist environmental aggressions. It even plumps out fine lines and prevents age spots. Drink 8 to 10 glasses of purified or filtered water every day, without fail.

✦ Get physical and get rest. Exercise exerts hormone-balancing effects on our skin. It also benefits the skin by increasing blood circulation, which provides nutrition to the skin cells; helps in expelling toxins; controls stress; and promotes deep, revitalizing sleep. Sleep time is when your entire body is busy regenerating, renewing, and rebuilding cellular tissue— which includes the healing of the hormone system.

YOUR SKIN CARE REGIMEN

When the foundation for our skin health has been laid by making the most of sunshine, fresh air, sleep, water, and food, it is time to turn to our skin care regimen. This includes five steps: protecting, cleansing, toning, moisturizing, and exfoliating. The steps can vary, depending on whether you're treating just your face or your entire body.

PROTECTING THE SKIN

Whatever you put on your skin plays a significant role in its long-term beauty. Inferior products can harm the skin by drying it out, clogging pores, irritating it, or causing allergic reactions. They can also affect our overall well-being. It's now proven that our skin absorbs the ingredients from personal-care products into the bloodstream. Many of these ingredients are proven to be hormone-disrupting as well as carcinogenic (cancer-causing).

Try to use the purest natural and organic products possible. Read ingredient labels and avoid anything with petrochemicals, synthetic fragrances, artificial colors, synthetic preservatives, harsh detergents, and alcohol. If in doubt, skin-care professionals can guide you to the purest skin-care treatments possible. In the meantime, remember that some of the purest and most nourishing skin-care treatments are close as your kitchen. We'll share a few of them here.

Regardless of the products you choose, always use a gentle massaging movement when manipulating your skin. Rough tugging, rubbing, or abrasive handling with your fingers, towels, tissues, or machines can damage your skin.

CLEANSING

Dry, aging, or damaged skin requires the gentlest cleansing agent possible; pH-balanced and nonsoap cleansers are preferred in the form of cleansing creams, lotions and milks. Look for botanical and certified organic ingredients and pure essential oils. High levels of antioxidants and anti-inflammatory ingredients will be of tremendous benefit for aging skin—including plant oils, vitamins, and minerals. Natural plant and nut oils cleanse, soften and protect the skin without clogging pores—like coconut oil, sweet almond oil, jojoba oil, and shea nut butter. They can replen-

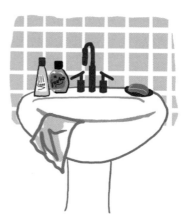

ish moisture without feeling oily. Used as cleansing oils, they can break down and dissolve makeup, dirt, and grime, while preserving the skin's protective lipid layer, or acid mantle. Oil traps residue and brings it to the surface, removing it when emulsified with warm water. Also consider the following:

Oatmeal Cleansing Mask

This mix is very hydrating, deep cleansing, and balancing for all skin types—but especially beneficial for mature, dry skin. Use on your whole body if desired (adjust ingredient amounts). The beta glucan in the oats penetrates to the deeper levels of the skin, eradicating fine lines and wrinkles. The almond oil imparts essential fatty acids, vitamins, and minerals, while honey is known for its humectancy (moisturizing effect). Use this cleansing mask at least once a week.

2 tablespoons ground oatmeal

½ tablespoon sweet almond oil

½ tablespoon honey

Thoroughly mix the ingredients together. Stroke over your face and neck in up-and-outward movements. Leave on for 20 minutes. Rinse thoroughly, then apply toner and moisturizer. Use this treatment once a week.

TONING

Dry, mature skin benefits from the use of a gentle toner. This clarifying liquid will firm and stimulate skin tissue, reduce pore size, and remove cleanser residue. There are many fine toners for dry and/ or mature skin available today that contain botanicals, herbs, and essential oils. Here's one you can make yourself.

Rose Water Toner

My favorite toner is rose water, a centuries-old secret for glowing skin. You can find rose water at natural-food stores as well as most Middle Eastern food stores. Or, try the following simple recipe, using rose otto essential oil— particularly beneficial for dry, mature skin.

4 drops rose otto essential oil

1 cup purified or filtered water

In a misting bottle, mix the essential oil and water and refrigerate. Shake before using. Mist over cleansed skin or dampen a cotton pad with the rose water and whisk over your skin in gentle upward, outward movements. You can do this over your face and body at intervals throughout the day.

Variation: Adding a few drops of jasmine essential oil to the rose water makes a very sensual body spray.

Hydrating lotions, creams, butters, and oils are valued for their humectancy (drawing moisture into the skin), emolliency (preserving moisture already existing in the skin), and lubrication (laying a protective layer on the outside of the skin). Moisturizers condition, repair, and protect. Look for products containing essential fatty acids, liposomes, peptides, or hyaluronic acid. Liposomes deliver nourishment to your skin's dermal layer, increasing the skin's internal water-binding capacity. Light vegetable or nut oils (sweet almond, avocado, hazelnut, rosehip, evening primrose—to name but a few) are particularly nutritive for aging skin. Use a small amount so it is absorbed quickly and gently apply to your face, neck, and entire body. This is particularly effective before going to bed at night. When applying to the face, do so in gentle upward and outward movements and gently pat with the pad of a fingertip around the eye area (outward along the top, inward along the bottom). Apply moisturizer to toned skin that is still damp to lock in valuable moisture.

The "Milky Way"

The professionals at the Flying Beauticians skin-care salon in San Francisco have come up with a home version of their two-step in-salon facial called "The Milky Way." It's divinely nourishing for the skin—the minerals in the chocolate have a calming effect, the polyphenols (antioxidants) thwart cell aging, and the decadent aroma releases feel-good endorphins. Lavender oil is calming, balancing, and moisturizing for the skin. The milk, egg yolk, and honey are moisturizing and nutritive. The lactic acid in milk has gentle exfoliating properties. Egg yolks are high in carotenoids (antioxidants). Consider omega-3 enriched eggs for an extra anti-inflammatory boost.

½ cup warm milk

1 teaspoon honey

1 teaspoon lavender essential oil

½ cup semisweet chocolate chips

1 tablespoon honey

1 egg yolk

In a bowl, mix together the milk, honey, and lavender oil. Apply to the face with your fingertips, using upward and outward movements. Leave on for 15 minutes. Rinse thoroughly.

In a separate bowl, heat the chocolate chips in the microwave just to the melting point. Mix in the honey and egg yolk. (Or, melt the chocolate in a double boiler over barely simmering water before adding the honey and egg yolk.) Slather this mixture onto your skin and leave for 10 minutes. Rinse off completely with warm water.

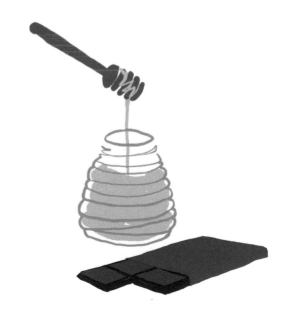

This technique removes the topmost dead layers of skin cells and debris to encourage better cell turnover, prevent clogged pores, and optimize the skin's moisture levels. Exfoliating is a vital step for aging skin, which can become dull, dry, and flaky if the top layer of cells is not removed regularly. Exfoliation may be done once a week. Many types of exfoliating products exist, from sugar scrubs to granular masks to alpha hydroxy acid lotions.

JUICY FRUITS

Alpha hydroxy acids, or AHAs, are natural exfoliants that help to remove dead surface cells, increase cell turnover, and plump up the lower layers of the skin to give a softer, moist look and feel. They've been shown to increase collagen in sun-damaged skin, and to reduce pore size, redness, blotchiness, and fine lines. AHAs are fruit acids that include glycolic acid from sugarcane, lactic acid from milk, tartaric acid from grapes, malic acid from apples, and citric acid from citrus fruits, among others. Many beauty products contain synthesized versions of these fruit acids and are available over the counter. You can also make your own.

Homemade AHA Skin Peel

Mix 1 teaspoon pure apple, lemon, grape, or papaya juice with a few drops of purified or filtered water and dab onto your cleansed skin with your fingers. Leave on for 5 to 10 minutes, then splash your face with plenty of water. Follow up with toner and moisturizer. This natural peel can be used once or twice a week.

MILK-BASED SKIN TREATMENTS

For the face and neck: Warm a little milk (heavy cream is better) and stir in an equal amount of honey. Spread this mixture on your face and neck. Leave on for 5 to 10 minutes and rinse with water.

A milk bath: Swirl about ½ cup dried milk into running warm bath water. Add a chamomile tea bag to the water. Sprinkle 4 to 6 drops of lavender essential oil under the running water when the tub is almost full. Leave the tea bag to soak along with you for 15 minutes. So calming, soothing, nourishing, and skin rejuvenative.

Enzyme Therapy Facial Treatment

The enzymes in many fruits can deep-cleanse and nourish the skin. Mash a small amount of banana, avocado, or pineapple and stir in a little honey. Gently apply to the face and neck with upward and outward movements. Leave on for 5 to 10 minutes and rinse off thoroughly with warm water.

TOO MUCH OF A GOOD THING

Don't overexfoliate. It can sensitize the skin and severely compromise the skin's barrier function. Once a week is often enough. Make sure to exfoliate at night, so your new skin isn't exposed to sunlight right away—new skin is more vulnerable to UV rays. And don't use more than one alpha hydroxy skin product per day. Consider using just a hydrating nighttime moisturizer with AHAs It's especially important to use an SPF 15 or higher sunscreen every day if you exfoliate and use skin treatments with AHAs; look for zinc- and titanium-based products. And if your skin is irritated by any treatment, calm it with a moisturizer that contains anti-inflammatory ingredients, like green tea. Again, count on a skin-care professional's expertise if you're not quite sure how to proceed with an exfoliation or AHA regimen.

MASSAGE

Massage stimulates blood and lymph flow throughout the body, making it a primary method for detoxification—including the excretion of excess hormones. Massage enhances our skin's cellular turnover, warms and strengthens connective tissue, and tones and lubricates the skin. It also reduces stress, increases endorphins, lifts depression, eases pain, lubricates joints, and can lower blood pressure. Whether your face, hands and feet, scalp, or entire body, massage your skin as often as possible.

Scented Massage Oil

Some of my favorite essential oils for skin-nourishing and anti-inflammatory benefits include chamomile, clary sage, orange blossom, geranium, lavender, peppermint, rosemary, sandalwood, ylang-ylang, and, last but not least, rose and rose hips. Depending on your personal preference, you can blend differ-ent oils in desired proportions. If you like, you can warm this massage oil to body temperature before applying it by placing the bottle in a bowl of very hot water for a few minutes.

You may use this oil for a massage ritual at any time of the day, whenever you have time and feel the need. It's especially helpful in the morning before showering, as it helps to center you for the day ahead, while at night it can be part of a relaxation ritual to encourage deep, restful sleep. Be fully pres-ent with yourself while performing this ritual. Any tension that you feel will melt away during this mood-enhancing practice.

15 drops essential oil of choice

2 tablespoons plant oil, such as sweet almond oil, avocado oil, hazelnut oil, evening primrose oil, or jojoba oil, or an organic body lotion

In a small bottle with a dispenser top, combine the essential oil and plant oil or lotion and shake to blend. Warm the oil if desired.

Work the oil between your hands, then massage into your skin, giving loving attention to the entire body or to specific areas that need special care. If doing a full-body massage, start at the scalp and gently massage from head to toe. Where appropriate, use upward and outward movements. At the very least, massage your scalp, hands, and feet.

INFLAMMATION EQUALS ACNE

Many skin problems are caused by inflammation. Quell the inflammation in the body, and you'll go a long way toward solving acne. This includes "inflamed" emotions.

Acne research shows that white bread, doughnuts (or any sugary food, for that matter), soft drinks, and other high-glycemic index foods are inflammatory, spiking blood sugar and insulin levels— which can incite overproduction of androgen (male) hormones and zits. Milk also creates problems, perhaps because of the high levels of artificial hormones in most milk. Drink organic milk if you drink it at all. Hormone replacement therapy can cause acne in certain individuals. When highly stressed, the body produces high levels of androgen hormones. This can stimulate the sebaceous glands to pump out more oil, resulting in acne. Achieve balance through stress-management techniques, diet, and physical activity. If you feel an eruption coming on, use tea tree essential oil: Place a drop on a cotton swab and touch it to the problem area; do not rinse off. Also, consider the following toner for its clarifying, purifying, and cooling effect on the skin. If your acne is severe, you should also see an experienced skin-care professional.

Acne-Clarifying Toner

3 to 5 drops peppermint, tea tree, lemon, or lemongrass essential oil

1 cup purified or filtered water

Combine the oil and water in a container with a lid. Shake thoroughly and let the mixture sit for 24 hours. Strain it through an organic paper coffee filter, pour into a clean misting bottle, and spray your face after cleansing or to simply freshen the skin at any point throughout the day.

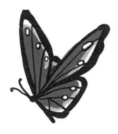

ROSACEA

Rosacea is quite prevalent in menopausal women. A red rash appears on the nose and cheeks that can be quite sensitive and burn. Other symptoms include broken capillaries and excessive oiliness in the T-zone. Rosacea is aggravated by many of the same things as acne. Stress and emotional upheaval—especially anger and anxiety—can bring on an episode. Overactivity, hot weather, tomatoes, seafood, preserved foods, sweets, and hot, sour, or fermented foods and beverages can all be triggers, along with antibiotics and harsh chemical peels, which oversensitize the skin.

Along with healing mind-body practices, make sure that you're getting the optimal levels of antioxidants and B vitamins. Drink water throughout the day—every hour on the hour. Consider drinking aloe vera juice in the morning.

Ultimately, all the lotions and potions for body care are secondary to the beautifying effects of a peaceful mind. "The best makeup is mind makeup," says T. Y. S. Lama Gangchen Rinpoche. "To make up the mind with inner peace actually makes us more beautiful."

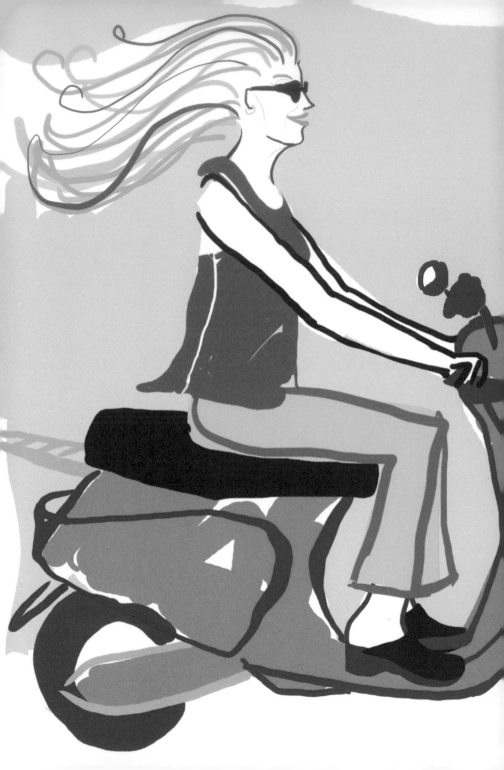

chapter 7

OUR CHANGING HAIR

A s we "bloom" into our most beautiful menopausal selves, hair thinning and textural changes can present challenges. Fine, thinning hair can make for less body and fullness. Hair can also become dry and lackluster, not only losing moisture but also its elasticity and ability to hold a curl. Most women desire some body in their hair, so we may resort to color and perms along with more styling products and tools to add fullness. The more we try to change it, the more fragile and duller it can become. We need to give our hair the greatest natural care possible—both inside and out. Stress management, optimizing your nutrition, regular physical activity, daily scalp massages, and loving care will provide beautifying and therapeutic value in caring for this most exquisite of fibers: our hair. ❡ We'll also look at the subject of superfluous hair growth. It can be a bit daunting to see a whisker or two pop up on your chin. Not to worry; there are many approaches to handling this situation, from the simplest to the more complex.

HAIR THINNING AND LOSS

Falling estrogen and excess testosterone levels contribute to the thinning and loss of head hair and unwanted hair growth elsewhere. Talk to your doctor to ensure that you've addressed hormonal imbalances, potential thyroid issues, or any other systemic reasons for hair thinning or loss.

One-third of menopausal women report noticeable hair loss or thinning. This can be emotionally devastating for many women. Not only does this hurt our self-esteem, but it's important to remember that hair, skin, and nail changes can be early warning signs for bodily ills. Noticing what's happening with your hair is an important part of self-care. Have hair and skin problems treated, as they can be indicators of disease. Hair loss due to falling estrogen levels is usually temporary and improves gradually, but other causes—like stress, poor diet, harsh hair care products and treatment, and other imbalances—aren't so fleeting and should be addressed.

THERAPIES FOR HEALTHY HAIR: FROM THE INSIDE OUT

Don't become obsessive about your hair if a small amount of thinning occurs; this may be part of the aging process for you. Look after yourself, accept yourself, love yourself, and everything else will fall into place. Here are some ways to make your hair look its best.

✦ Begin by being honest about how well you're doing at managing stressors, because they can be a major factor in hormonal balance and overall health. Practice forgiveness and emotional cleansing as often as needed. Anger and its evil cousin, rage, are associated with higher levels of testosterone.

✦ Look for dietary causes of hair loss and thinning. An organic, whole-foods, protein-rich diet is essential. (Hair is about 97 percent protein and 3 percent moisture.) This will shield you from pesticide residues as well as chemical, antibiotic, and hormone additives. Greatly reduce or eliminate refined sugar and high-carbohydrate foods like white sugar and white flour products. These can create elevated blood glucose levels and potential insulin sensitivity, which is linked to hair loss. Also limit coffee, saturated and trans fats, and salt.

✦ Make sure that you're getting all your vitamins, minerals, and antioxidants. Take a high-quality multivitamin daily that includes 100 percent of the recommended daily allowance for hair-healthy vitamins such as A, B, C and E. Other important nutrients are folic acid, niacin, pantothenic acid, panthenol, calcium, magnesium, copper, zinc, selenium, boron, and iron. Foods rich in silicon (green and red peppers, potato skins, and sprouts) will strengthen hair. Sea vegetables, like kelp, are also good for the hair. Kelp adds iodine to the diet, which is important in manufacturing thyroid hormones.

✦ Drink those 8 glasses of purified or filtered water every day! Your hair's resilience and shine depends on it.

✦ Get your recommended daily allowance of essential fatty acids. Take GLA (gamma linolenic acid) in the form of black currant, evening primrose, or borage oils. Holistic doctors recommend 500 mg twice a day. Increase your consumption of omega-3 essential fatty acids (found in fatty fish, walnuts, and flax-seeds), whether from food or supplemental oils. Consider high-lignan flaxseed oil, cod liver oil, or fish oil containing vitamin D. In six to eight weeks you should see greatly improved hair and skin. Omega-3 EFA's will also help boost immunity and soothe inflammation.

✦ Ginkgo biloba has a dynamic effect on mental sharpness and memory because it increases blood flow to the brain; for the same reason, it nourishes the scalp.

+ Dong quai can be helpful for thinning hair. The herb contains substances similar to estrogen, which can counter the effect of male hormones on further hair thinning. Try it in teas, tinctures, or capsules.

+ Scalp massage is very helpful for stimulating blood flow to the scalp, thus feeding nutrients to the hair follicles. It also keeps the scalp flexible and encourages cellular turnover.

Scalp Massage

Aside from your nutritional intake, keeping the scalp as flexible as possible is your number-one practice for healthy hair growth. A well-tended scalp can, over time, age-proof our hair. As we age, the scalp begins to thin and tighten, which affects hair growth and appearance. Scalp massage relieves stress and stimulates blood flow and oil production, thereby feeding the hair nutrients and giving it luster, pliability, and protection. Scalp massage can keep hair follicles young, extending the life span of a hair strand by years. In a study published in *Archives of Dermatology*, researchers showed that a daily scalp massage using certain essential oils mixed with plant oil was highly effective at stimulating hair growth.

I'm a huge proponent of daily massage, with or without essential oils or plant oils. Just place your fingertips on your scalp at any time of the day and gently massage or "rake" (move your fingertips back and forth over your scalp) for a few minutes. Remember, a healthy, stimulated scalp = healthy hair.

An Aromatherapy Scalp Treatment

This is a powerhouse protein and moisturizing treatment for the scalp and hair. Use it before your morning shower, or leave on overnight (cover your pillow with a towel).

Note: This treatment is quite safe; however, if you are pregnant or have high blood pressure, diabetes, or epilepsy, check with your doctor before using this aromatherapy treatment.

> 2 drops thyme essential oil
>
> 2 drops cedarwood essential oil
>
> 3 drops lavender essential oil
>
> 3 drops rosemary essential oil
>
> 1 ½ tablespoons plant oil, such as sweet almond,
>   jojoba, or sesame

In a small bottle with a spout, combine the essential oils and plant oil. Shake to blend. Warm the oil if desired. Massage into your scalp for several minutes, using your fingertips to make small rotary movements from the front hairline back toward the crown, the side temple areas toward the center back occipital area, and from behind the ears across the nape of the neck. Work the oil through the hair lengths as well.

Cover your hair with a shower cap or warm towel. Leave on for 30 minutes or longer. Wet the hair and then shampoo.

To remedy hair loss/thinning, do this aromatherapy massage every day, initially for several weeks, then taper off to once a week (though you may not want to!).

THE HOLISTIC APPROACH TO HAIR CARE

Many techniques, tools, and products can take their toll on the hair. Mass-marketed personal care products can expose us to a large number of toxic ingredients. Instead, look for organic plant extracts, plant oils, natural and organic essential oils, and whole-food derivatives. They do for the hair and scalp what they do for the body, providing a high level of antioxidants, vitamins and minerals, enzymes, amino acids, essential fatty acids, phytosterols, and natural sugars to your hair and scalp. They will balance, strengthen, hydrate, relax, stimulate, and detoxify your hair and scalp.

If you want to color or permanent-wave your hair, work with a hair-care professional. Chemical processes alter the hair's natural structure, which can weaken the hair. If you do color or wave your hair, apply a light protective application of a high-antioxidant, anti-inflammatory plant oil like sesame or coconut oil onto the scalp before proceeding (don't massage the scalp, just gently stroke the oil onto the scalp with your fingertips).

Hair is made of protein and moisture—therefore, as our hair becomes more fragile or dry, protein and moisturizing treatments are essential to strengthen and hydrate it, keeping it resilient and shiny. Become a label reader. If the ingredient list is a long, indiscernible list of chemicals, think twice about using. Many wonderful small companies are creating some very pure nontoxic lines of hair and skin care products.

YOUR HAIR-CARE REGIMEN

HAIR CLEANSING

Many hair experts recommend shampooing fine, dry hair about three times a week, rinsing well on the in-between days and putting a dollop of conditioner through the hair as needed. (Women who use a lot of heavy/firm-hold styling products, however, may want to shampoo more often.) Use gentle pH-balanced and sulfate-free shampoos, preferably organic ones. This prevents the stripping of protein and natural oils from the hair and scalp. Make doubly sure to massage the scalp on the days you don't shampoo to keep it flexible, as shampooing itself is a great way to "exercise" the scalp, stimulating hair growth. After shampooing, rinse, rinse, rinse to remove all shampoo residue from the hair and scalp.

If you color your hair, faithfully use a shampoo and conditioner for color-treated hair. Your hair color's longevity and vibrancy depends on it.

STRENGTHEN YOUR HAIR TREATMENTS

No matter what kind of shampoo, conditioner, or massage oil you use, you can pump up the benefits by mixing organic ingredients into it. For instance, you can add a few drops of rosemary essential oil to your shampoo or massage oil to stimulate blood circulation and hair growth and smooth the cuticle, creating incredible shine (lavender, orange blossom, peppermint, and other essential oils will do the same). Or, add a beaten egg to your shampoo or conditioner. Milk and yogurt are also high in protein and can strengthen weak hair. Use penetrating natural conditioners like aloe vera or honey, or plant oils like jojoba, coconut, avocado, rose hip, or sweet almond oil to moisturize your hair and scalp. Rinse or shampoo out as needed.

HAIR RINSES

After shampooing, it's helpful to use a rinse to remove any shampoo residue, return the hair/scalp to its natural acid balance, and moisturize. This is especially true if you've used oil as a pre-shampoo treatment on your hair or scalp.

✦ Steep 2 tablespoons dried herbs in 1 cup boiling water. Let cool, then strain. Put into a bottle with spout and use after shampooing and towel-drying your hair. Herb choices: Panax ginseng replenishes moisture, giving the hair flexibility and sheen. Chamomile is emollient, anti-inflammatory, and shine-enhancing. Lavender will smoothen and add shine to the hair. Nettles add fullness.

✦ You can also add 3 to 5 drops of essential oil for its aromatic and therapeutic properties (try geranium, jasmine, lavender, orange blossom, sandalwood, or ylang-ylang).

✦ You can also add any type of vinegar: apple cider, plum, or raspberry to your final rinse water. It restores the hair's natural pH balance and seals the cuticle, creating wonderful shine. Use 1 tablespoon to 1 cup of water.

CONDITIONERS

If you don't use the pre-shampoo oil massage, use a daily conditioner. Depending on hair type, you may also want to use a leave-in conditioner on towel-dried hair. These conditioners are particularly good for overly porous, dry hair. Some of them even add body to the hair, so that you don't have to add additional styling products. Also consider working a few drops of camellia oil through the hair after towel drying to condition the hair and serve as a hair dressing.

DEEP PROTEIN AND MOISTURIZING TREATMENTS FOR DRY HAIR/SCALP

The aromatherapy hair/scalp massage on page 91 will serve as a deep protein/moisturizing treatment when used once a week, but there are many marvelous hair and scalp treatments on the market. Or, make your own. They'll soothe dry, brittle, damaged hair and make it feel silky, lustrous and full.

✦ Make a hair smoothie out of a small, ripe banana, 1 tablespoon honey, and 1 tablespoon sweet almond oil. Mix together and work the mixture through your hair and scalp. Leave on for 30 minutes, and then rinse thoroughly.

✦ Mash a ripe avocado, mix with 1 tablespoon jojoba oil, and massage into hair and scalp. Cover with a shower cap and/or a warm towel and leave on for 30 minutes before shampooing as usual.

+ Blackstrap molasses is a great treatment for damaged hair. Massage some into your hair, cover with a shower cap and/or warm towel, and allow it to remain on for as long as possible before rinsing.

Egg Yolk and Walnut Oil Deep Treatment

I use this at least once a month. The results are amazing: shiny, thick, and luxuriant feeling hair. It's better than any store-bought treatment. Adjust amounts depending on hair length and density.

> 2 egg yolks
>
> 1 tablespoon walnut oil
>
> 2 drops essential oil of choice, such as lemon, jasmine, rose, sandalwood, or rosemary

In a small bowl, beat the egg yolks with the walnut oil and essential oils. Massage the mixture through your hair and scalp. Cover with a shower cap and/or a warm towel and leave on for up to 1 hour, if possible. To remove, rinse well with warm water, then shampoo well and rinse.

SENSE OF STYLE

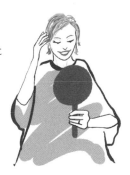

The hair's density and textural changes that come with age can be addressed with the right haircut and style. Lightweight styling products are helpful for volumizing the hair. Work closely with an experienced holistic hair stylist who will honor your hair type in the cutting/styling process.

IT'S ALL ABOUT THE BODY!

To give your hair more body, consider the following:

+ Get a haircut every 6 to 8 weeks to keep the ends fresh.

✦ Use lightweight non- or low-alcohol volumizing products—
including nonaerosol hair spray. (Alcohol dries out the hair and
is especially damaging when your hair is exposed to sunlight.)

✦ Use natural-bristle brushes; they're less damaging to the hair.

✦ Let your hair dry naturally whenever possible. Heat is the
number-one source of hair damage. If you must use a hair
dryer, use the lowest setting (check out the new ionic dryers).
Consider a diffuser attachment to spread the air over a larger
area. Also, keep the dryer in constant motion, rather than
focusing the blowing air on one area at a time. Avoid curling
irons, if possible—instead, use round brushes to add fullness
or bevel edges after the hair is almost dry. Or, use Velcro
rollers in spot areas where fullness is desired.

✦ Massage a light- to medium-hold styling product through your
hair and comb it into your desired style. Let dry naturally, or
use a diffuser, then brush, comb, or run your fingers through
your hair. Spray with a light-hold non-aerosol hairspray if
desired. Work a few drops of a shiner product (or camellia oil)
into the palms of your hands and sweep them over the surface
of your hair or massage thoroughly through all the hair to
impart a radiant shine.

✦ Add a revitalizing lift to your hair by tossing your head forward
and massaging the entire scalp area. Lightly mist with hair
spray on the underneath lengths if desired. Lift your head up
and place the hair with your fingers. This is an instant hair
bodifier!

HAIR, HAIR, GO AWAY, COME BACK ANOTHER DAY

Many women are distressed at the signs of hairs sprouting on their
face (as well as other body parts). Not to worry, there are lots of

ways to go fuzz-free. Having been assured by your doctor that your androgen hormones are not out of whack, you may proceed assuredly to pluck, razor, or lighten away.

First, buy the very best tweezer that money can buy from a beauty supply store. A tweezer of this type will make tweezing effortless *and* painless. Pluck in the direction of hair growth. This remedy may need to be done every few days or once every week or two—it depends on the fineness or coarseness of the hair (and over time, these hairs may take much longer to come back or not come back at all).

Razoring superfluous hair away is an option for treating areas like the lipline. Purchase a delicate little razor wand, specifically made for a woman's special needs, at your local drugstore. Use short, feathery strokes in the direction of the hair growth on freshly cleansed and lubricated skin (and apply a dab of almond, olive, or sesame oil). The pores will be open, and hair more easily removed without irritation. Repeat as needed. There are also battery operated facial-hair removers, like tiny electric razors, widely available. The myth that shaving makes hair grow in thicker is just that—a myth. Razoring hair away is best for fine- to medium-texture hair. If the hair is coarse, you may prefer to tweeze or wax, in order to remove the hair from the root.

For small and large areas alike, home waxing kits are available. Waxing kits come with handy-dandy prewaxed strips. Or, see a professional to have waxing services done. Over time, waxing will greatly diminish or end hair growth, while electrolysis and laser hair-removal methods will banish those hairs for good. There is also a technique called "threading" that is quickly gaining ground in beauty salons and spas. A length of thread is used to whisk the hair out from the root. It is quick and painless.

There is one other option for facial hair. For fine- to medium-texture hair, you may choose to use store-bought hair lighteners.

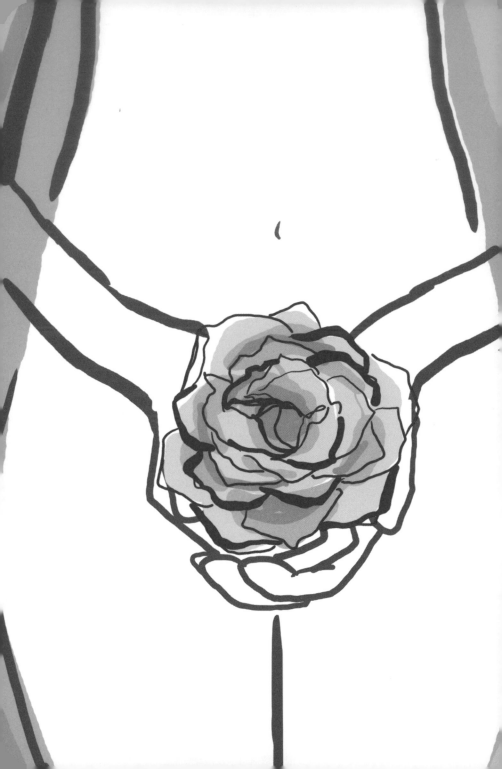

chapter 8

GO WITH THE FLOW, OR STAYING LUBRICATED INSIDE AND OUT

Hormonal change can bring menstrual, vaginal, and urinary changes. The menstrual cycle can become quite irregular, as can its duration and intensity—particularly during perimenopause. Urinary incontinence and weak pelvic muscles may also become more prevalent during this time. In this chapter, we'll soothe the way with balancing therapies and remedies.

VAGINAL HEALTH

A decline in estrogen can create vaginal dryness and irritation. Aging truly can be a matter of "drying up." To stay as "juicy" as possible, both outside and inside, try the following:

✦ Make sure you're getting enough essential fatty acids (omega-3s from fatty fish, fish oil, evening primrose oil, or flaxseed) in your diet; they can be very helpful in staying lubricated.

✦ Stay well hydrated. Eat water-packed foods (lots of fresh, organic fruits and veggies). As mentioned previously, drinking 8 to 10 glasses of water every day helps prevent the drying of the skin and the mucous membranes. Sip a bit of water every hour on the hour.

✦ Use nonhormonal vaginal lubricants to alleviate dryness and nourish vaginal tissues. Vitamin E oil, aloe vera gel, or olive, sesame, coconut, or sweet almond oil can be used to moisturize your vaginal area. (Plant oils can break down the latex in condoms, so beware that combination.) Products that contain vitamin E, black cohosh, and wild yam are also nourishing, safe, and healing to the vaginal tissue. Try mixing slippery elm powder and aloe vera gel into a paste and inserting into your vagina at night to relieve dryness. Or try store-bought natural, organic lubricants (without preservatives such as parabens or propylene glycol, please!).

✦ Regular intercourse or self-love (yes, masturbation!) is also beneficial, because it boosts estrogen levels and increases blood flow to the vaginal tissues. Use one of the suggested lubricants above, and you're golden. Regular aerobic exercise also promotes blood circulation to the pelvic area.

- Use pure, nontoxic, organic body washes to cleanse the genital area. It is simply not necessary to use harsh, alkaline deodorant soaps in this area.

- Wear clothing made from natural fibers, especially cotton, so that the skin can breathe, thus decreasing the chance of vaginal infections. Wear loose, comfortable organic cotton or silk undergarments.

THE VAGINA MONOLOGUES

Don't be shy when it comes to talking about vaginal health! Consider exclusively using organic tampons and pads. Why? The chlorine byproduct dioxin—a chemical that acts like estrogen in the body—occurs in the chlorine-treated rayon fibers that are in some brands of tampons. Dioxin collects in our fat cells, affecting hormone balance. Organic tampons and pads are made of material whitened with hydrogen peroxide instead of chlorine. They're also made with 100 percent organically grown cotton. When we remove a tampon, some fibers remain inside the vagina. In the United States, more than one billion tons of pesticides and herbicides are sprayed on cotton crops every year. Some of these residues may taint tampons. With organic materials, you're not exposing delicate vaginal walls to residual pesticides, herbicides, growth regulators, or defoliants. These can function as hormone disrupters, damage the nervous system, and even lead to cancer with long-term exposure.

At a time when our hormones are potentially askew anyway, we shouldn't add to our body's burden, don't you agree?

URINARY INCONTINENCE

There are many causes for urinary incontinence, or "leakage": a reduction in estrogen, weak pelvic muscles, urinary tract infections, and lower collagen levels are just a few (collagen holds the body tissues together). An irritated bladder can bring on the urge, or worse, prevent us from "holding it." Bladder irritants may include diet soda, citrus, chocolate, and alcohol.

DON'T BE A DRIP—SQUEEZE THOSE KEGELS

Kegel exercises can prevent urine leakage. They also condition and tone the pelvic floor muscles, increase blood circulation to this area, and help in keeping the tissues healthy and moist. An additional benefit? Enhanced lovemaking.

✦ Tighten the pubococcygeus, also known as the PC muscles, for 10 seconds, then relax. If you're contracting your PC muscles, you'll feel like you're trying to stop yourself from urinating. Repeat 10 times. Remember to breathe. Inhale on the contraction, exhale on the release.

✦ Do this several times during the day. You can do Kegel exercises almost anytime: while waiting at red lights or in line at the store, while listening to music, preparing a meal, or doing any beautifying ritual. But whatever you do, do them. I do them while in yoga's "Goddess" pose (a great pose for "opening" and bringing energy into the hip/pelvic area): lying on my back with my arms out to the side, bottoms of my feet together, and knees dropped down to the sides.

IN CONTROL WITH YOGA

Yoga has a wide variety of postures that help to tighten the pelvic floor muscles. Here is a particularly effective one:

THE MOVING CAT POSE

This yoga pose strengthens your PC muscles. And you get the extra bonus of breathing deeply, releasing tension in the lower back, and flexing the entire spine.

✦ Kneel on all fours with your knees underneath your hipbones and your wrists one hand's distance forward of the shoulders (to alleviate pressure on the wrists).

✦ Gently pull your belly in and draw your shoulders back, bringing your spine parallel to the floor.

✦ On the inhale, flex your spine by lifting your breastbone/head up and forward, rounding your belly toward the floor. As you do this, gently draw your tailbone toward your heels to protect your lower spine.

✦ As you exhale, round your spine upward toward the sky like a Halloween cat; look down, drawing your pelvis toward the floor and your lower belly strongly inward while contracting the PC muscles.

✦ At the peak of your exhale, sit back on your heels (with your tailbone drawn toward the heels), keeping your arms fully extended in front of you. Inhale and rise to the starting position.

✦ Repeat this sequence 3 times, working up to 6. Do at least once a day.

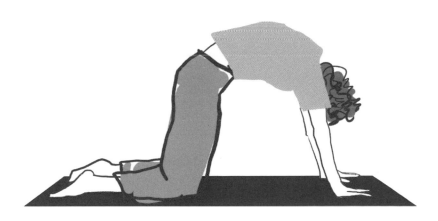

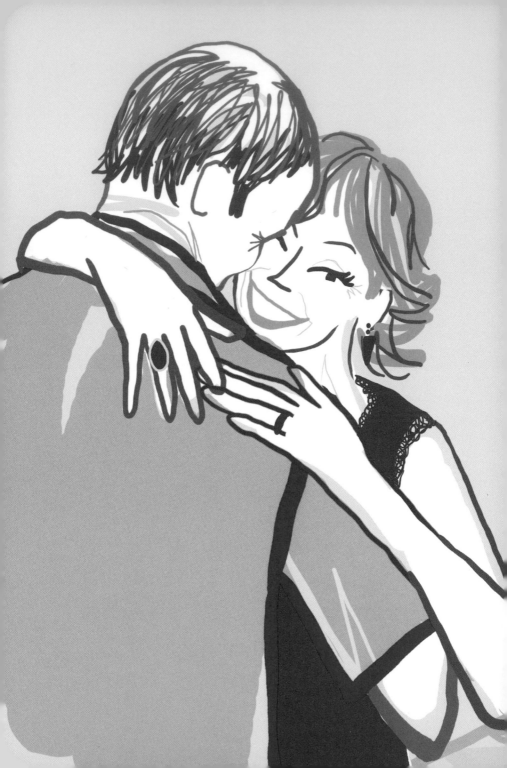

chapter 9

SENSUAL HEALING: ENHANCING OUR LIBIDO

If we're seeking to rediscover our sexuality during this phase of life, looking inward and reflecting on who we are, why we're here, and what would make us truly happy becomes a valuable practice. See your desires very clearly, visualize them, and give them a voice. ❡ You may have heard the expression, "The most important sexual organ is the mind." However, menopausal sensations like fatigue, mood swings, and bodily changes can shut us off from our sensual self (30 to 40 percent of postmenopausal women have diminished libidos). Recovering sexual desire takes commitment. It's very easy in today's stressful and time-starved world to let sexual satisfaction fall by the wayside. ❡ It's time to renew this wonderful relationship with your sexual self. We know that estrogen and testosterone imbalance can be a sexual saboteur, along with psychological or body-image problems, relationship problems, sexual abuse (23 percent of all women have been sexually abused), certain medications, chronic pain or disease, and stress incontinence. Discuss your situation with your doctor or a well-qualified therapist. Once you've eliminated the more serious concerns, you'll find that there are many effective options for women who want to restore the spark in their lives.

HAVE THE RIGHT ATTITUDE

Loss of libido is a problem with many solutions. It's no one's "fault." In a committed relationship, what affects one partner has an impact on the other. This is a time to come together and communicate openly and lovingly. The best aphrodisiac in the world is a partner who is warm, nurturing, communicative, and willing to explore options that work for both partners. Everyone has her or his own needs and desires in regard to being pleasured. But they need to be shared. Despite changes in hormone levels and libido, there are ways to work around them and maintain sexual activity. Your attitude may be your most valuable asset. Some testimonials: One friend says that she enjoys her sex life more now than ever. Why? Because "I'm lucky enough to have a partner who knows what I like, and I'm not afraid to tell him what I need." Hugely important!

And this: "With our kids all gone, we're alone for the first time in thirty years. I now realize that every moment holds the potential for foreplay—every glance, every touch, every conversation. Even our arguments. It's true—make-up sex can be the best!" These two know the value of flirting—a great aphrodisiac!

And last but not least: "There's nothing wrong with my libido that a little TLC from my husband won't fix. It has nothing to do with menopause." Wow!

ENHANCING SEXUAL DESIRE

Whatever the reason for a lessened sex drive, following are some healthy, gentle ways to enhance your desires and reconnect with this beautiful experience.

✦ Set a mood. Indulge all the senses in the bedroom, with massage oil (sensual touch is one of the ultimate turn-ons), your favorite CDs (Marvin Gaye does it every time!), intimate lighting, a scented candle, an aromatherapy diffuser or fragrant mist sprayed through the room, fresh flowers, a beautifully arranged platter of finger foods, chocolate, wine, and fresh sheets—silky satin, fuzzy flannel, high-thread count, whatever turns you on.

✦ Certain aromas conjure love—even downright lust. Research has shown a connection between sexual arousal in some women and the sweet smell of Good & Plenty candy, baby powder, pumpkin pie, and lavender oil! All of these fragrances caused measurable increases in vaginal blood flow, a known marker of sexual arousal. Researchers theorize that certain scents trigger mood-lightening happy memories, and that these scents may also act on brain chemicals that control mood. Also consider these aromas for their aphrodisiac effect: cardamom, cinnamon, ginger, jasmine, neroli (orange blossom), patchouli, rose, geranium, sandalwood, vanilla, and ylang-ylang. These are available in the form of spices, essential oils, incense, candles, commercially prepared lotions and potions, and more.

✦ If you snore a lot, seek treatment from your doctor. Ask him or her to do a sleep study to determine if you have obstructive sleep apnea. This condition, where the airway becomes blocked during sleep and breathing briefly halts, can cause snoring. It is a potentially dangerous condition. It suppresses hormone functions and diminishes oxygen levels in the bloodstream. Researchers found improvements in sexual response after sleep apnea was successfully treated.

If sleep apnea is not a problem, consider the following general recommendations: If overweight, try to slim down. Obesity contributes to snoring. Sleep on your side, not your back. Sometimes, this alone is enough to solve the problem. Try adding an extra pillow; elevating your head may relieve snoring. There are "snoring" strips that you can purchase—they adhere to the bridge of the nose, and they hold the sides of the nasal passages open wider then normal to increase air flow. Also, avoid eating within two hours of bedtime. Minimize your consumption of salt/salty foods. If sodium levels are high, potassium levels may be low, and low levels of potassium are associated with snoring. Avoid alcohol, or if you do drink, limit to two hours away from bedtime. Alcohol causes a snorer to sleep more heavily and snore more loudly. Also avoid taking antihistamines, tranquilizers, or any other type of medication that depresses the central nervous system. There are many other treatments for snoring, including nutritional supplements, herbs, and homeopathy.

✦ Herbs like maca and damiana can enhance sexual desire, pleasure, and performance. They may be taken in tea, tincture, and capsule form, and in synergistic blends with other herbs. Many other libido-boosting herbs are available; however, these two are the most commonly used. Do research before using, as there are contraindications with certain health conditions and medications.

✦ The fastest way to spruce up your sex life? Toys! Vibrators have gone from déclassé to a must-have accessory. Whether you're single or part of a couple, take my advice: Get a toy. You have every right to fully pleasure yourself. If your libido is challenged, this could be the perfect therapy for getting back on track. Regular, ecstatic orgasm is one of the most healing and profound therapies. And while you're toy shopping, on the Internet or locally, make sure to include some of the wonderful products that are available to enhance your lovemaking— lubes, balms, dusts, lotions, and potions.

Sensual Aromatherapy Room Mist

This sensual mist can be used in your bedroom and during or after your bath to enhance your lovemaking mood. Try combining rose and vanilla; sandalwood and vanilla; patchouli and ylang-ylang; or geranium, lavender, and neroli. Use fewer drops of the essential oils, making the spray more dilute, if it will be used on the skin.

10 to 30 drops of your favorite essential oil(s)

1 teaspoon vodka (to help disperse the essential oils)

½ cup purified or filtered water

In a 4-ounce mist bottle, combine the oil(s) and vodka and shake well. Add the water and shake well again. Mist in the air, on clothes, bed linens, hair, light bulbs, and so on.

Decadent Chocolate Sauce

An opulent dessert topping—for you or your lover. Mother Nature's favorite sweet is a welcome addition to any sexual repertoire. A luscious aphrodisiac and stimulant, it raises endorphins. You may want to consider using sheets that are specifically designated for your chocolate lovemaking escapades.

7 ounces bittersweet chocolate, chopped

½ cup organic sugar

¾ cup purified or filtered water

1 tablespoon butter

Flavoring to taste: almond or vanilla extract; chocolate, hazelnut, or fruit liqueur; etc.

In a double boiler over barely simmering water, combine the chocolate, sugar, and water. Stir constantly until the chocolate is melted. Remove from the heat and stir in the butter and flavoring.

SWEATING IS SEXY

The overall health-boosting benefits of exercise are well proven. Included among them are improved sexual functioning and better sexual self-esteem. A research study showed that 88 percent of women and 69 percent of men who worked out four to five days a week rated their sexual performance from above average to *way* above average. In addition, researchers said that these individuals "perceived themselves as more confident and sexually desirable." They also determined that regular exercise can help to prevent the decline in sexual performance and satisfaction that often accompanies aging.

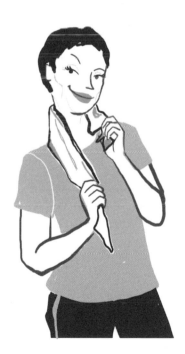

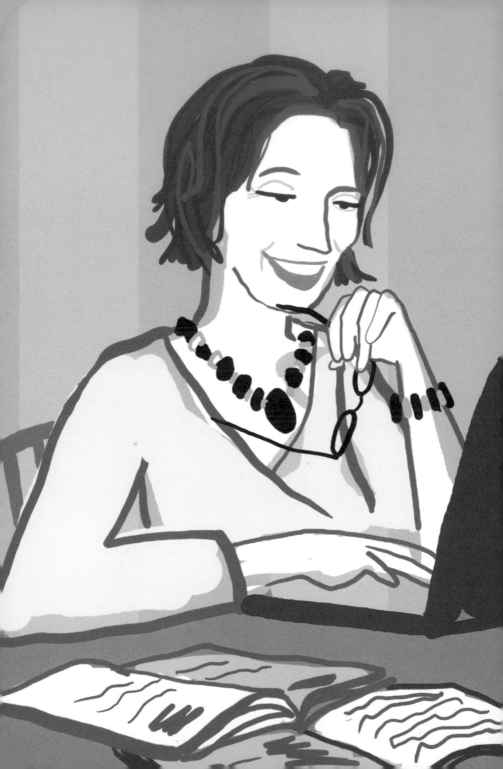

PART THREE

Primary Health Care

Three of the major health-care concerns linked with menopause are heart disease, bone health, and (breast) cancer. Although we will not venture into the realm of medical treatment here, you will find some sage advice for making a beneficial connection with your doctor, ideally a holistic doctor who works within the CAM system (complementary and alternative medicine), or works with "integrative medicine." None of us should have our heads in the proverbial sand when it comes to primary health-care issues. Awareness is power when serving as our own wellness advocate—and perhaps supporting and sharing with other women as well.

As we progress through menopause, estrogen levels fluctuate and fall; however, cumulative exposure over a lifetime, combined with lifestyle factors in the present, can create imbalances that if left uncorrected can impact our health profile post menopause. With a diminished amount of estrogen circulating through the body after menopause, our risk for heart disease and osteoporosis may rise, while excess estrogen and/or progesterone may contribute to the occurrence of breast cancer. High cumulative exposure to estrogen over our lifetime can factor into the equation here, whether because of early onset of menstruation, not getting pregnant or breastfeeding, having short and more frequent menstrual cycles, or experiencing menopause past the age of fifty-five. It is recommended that you confer with your doctor in determining your own unique hormonal profile. In this section, you'll find helpful suggestions to guide you.

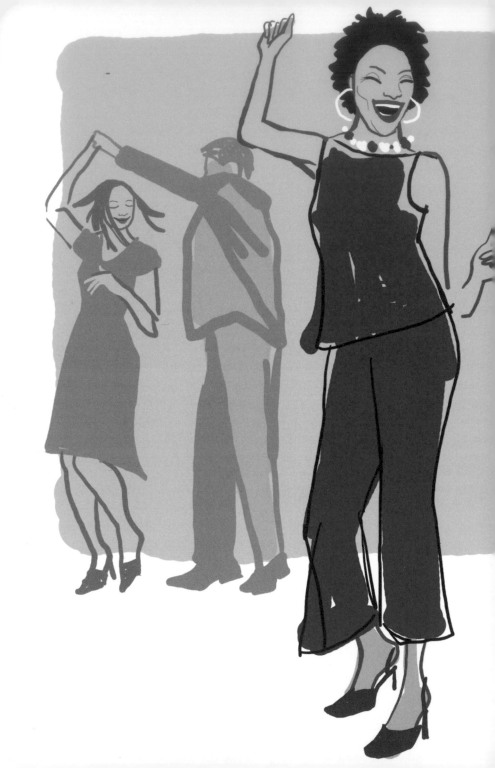

chapter 10

THE ESSENTIALS OF BONE HEALTH

Which one of us wouldn't want to enjoy spectacular musculoskeletal health into our final years? The possibility is real, if you put some safeguards in place. Osteoporosis is a bone-weakening disease: a condition that causes bones to become porous and brittle. Those who have osteoporosis have a significantly increased risk of fracturing bones. Postmenopausal women are particularly susceptible to osteoporosis, but the seeds of this condition are planted long before, a result of both genetics and lifestyle. Our "peak bone mass" is generally around age thirty and begins to decline after this. After menopause, we can lose 1 to 5 percent of our bone density yearly (due to diminishing estrogen and its bone-protective qualities). All the more reason to put the brakes on bone loss as soon as possible. ⟡ If you're at an increased risk for osteoporosis, be proactive and ask your physician to do a bone-density test. Early attention from your doctor, plus the tips in this chapter, will help keep your bones strong.

PHYSICAL ACTIVITY
BUILDS BONES

Experts say that physical activity is the single most important influence on bone density. This is a very important factor for both aging women and men—especially for women who are susceptible to osteoporosis. Weight-bearing exercise maintains bones, slows bone mineral loss, preserves muscle strength, and boosts balance. Lifting weights, dancing, walking, skipping rope, climbing stairs, strengthening yoga postures—will all aid bone density.

PUMP IT UP!

What's the best bone-saving, density-building workout? Strength or weight training. Research shows that women who did strength training twice a week for one year actually gained bone density versus a control group who did no training and lost bone density. In addition, increased muscle mass from lifting weights will torch more calories and help control blood sugar (helpful for that creeping weight gain as we get older!), while strong muscles make everyday activities simpler. Strength training is proven to help us maintain better balance. Then there is the toning benefit for the muscles, which equals overall shapeliness. Invest in a basic dumbbell set and a beginners' weight-training DVD. Or, sign up for a weight-training class through your local park district or gym. You can also check the Internet for weight-training lessons, or splurge on a personal trainer. So start pumping it up, ladies!

YOGA'S DOG POSES

My pooch, Luna, does Downward- and Upward-Facing Dog to perfection. We humans could learn from the great enjoyment that our pets get from stretching. These postures release overall tension, increase flexibility, lengthen and strengthen the entire spinal column and the abdominals, and strengthen and lubricate the muscles, joints, tendons, and bones of the hands, arms, shoulders, back, ankles, and more. They'll stimulate our bones to retain calcium, and thus are very helpful in preventing bone deterioration and loss—and they may actually stimulate bone growth. They will also strengthen and shape muscles you didn't know you had!

Downward Dog is also an inversion posture that gives the heart a break from gravity. In Upward Dog, the chest is opened while lifting the entire body off the floor. In both postures, the body is supported by the hands and feet. Try each one of these postures singularly, and then try combining them. You may only be able to do one sequence of this combination at first, but as your strength increases you will be able to build up to 10 repetitions or more.

Downward-Facing Dog

+ Kneel on all fours on a yoga mat. Your knees should be underneath your hipbones, your hands one hand's distance forward of the shoulders (and shoulder-width apart). Your fingers are spread open wide, with your hands pressing into the mat.

+ Firm your inner thighs inward and back and draw your tailbone toward your heels. Curl your toes into the floor. On an exhale, lift your buttocks toward the sky, pressing into the floor through your hands. If your heels don't reach the floor, that's okay; with practice, they will.

+ Let your head hang between your arms. Keep your buttocks extending up toward the sky while reaching deeply into the earth through your hands. Breathe smoothly and naturally for several breaths.

+ Release your body back down to all fours. Sit back on your heels, while lowering your torso and head toward the floor into Child's Pose, a wonderfully restorative posture.

+ If you feel pressure in your wrists while doing Down Dog, roll up a towel and place it under the back heel of the wrist to alleviate excessive pressure.

✦ Lie face-down on a yoga mat. Position your hands with fingers spread on either side of the chest, just below your shoulders. Keep your elbows close to your body. Place your feet hip-width apart, with the top of the feet firmly planted into the floor. Firm your thighs and buttocks and gently draw your tailbone toward your heels.

✦ On an inhalation, lift your body off the floor, straightening your arms and opening through the chest. Keep your shoulders drawn down and back. Look forward or slightly up, keeping your neck long and relaxed.

✦ Try to keep your pubic bone and legs off the floor. Press down through your hands as you keep your body lifting away from the floor. And remember to breathe!

✦ On an exhalation, lower your body to the floor. Great upper-body stengthening here! Place your arms by your sides and turn your head (rest on your cheek) to the right for a couple of breaths, then turn your head to the other side for a couple of breaths. You may also go into Child's Pose if you'd like.

To combine, begin with Downward-Facing Dog, then fluidly move directly into Upward-Facing Dog. You may do both postures to an exhalation and inhalation. Or you may take several breaths in each pose before moving into the next one.

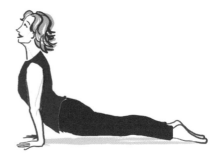

BOOST YOUR BONES

Eating calcium-rich foods like leafy green vegetables, low-fat dairy products, and calcium-fortified orange juice and cereal, along with adequate vitamin D intake can prevent loss of bone mass. Vitamin D promotes calcium absorption. (It's recommended that women ingest 1,000 to 1,200 mg of calcium a day before menopause and 1,500 mg post menopause.)

Vitamin B_{12} is also proving to be significant in the prevention of osteoporosis. The recommended dietary allowance for adults is 2.4 micrograms daily. Food sources include meats, eggs, and dairy, along with fortified cereals.

And do "bone up" on isoflavone-rich foods, such as soy. A study with more than twenty-four thousand postmenopausal women showed that those who ate the most soy in the group (13 g daily) slashed their risk of future bone breaks or fractures by 36 percent (that's 2 cups of soy milk a day). A cautionary note here: See the section on breast health and soy consumption (page 134). If breast cancer is a risk for you, based on family history, then you may need to dial down the soy consumption. When in doubt, get your phytoestrogens from a widely varied diet.

"Soy Nutty" Granola   MAKES 6 CUPS, SERVES 12

This is not only a great breakfast but a great snack after working out, because of its high protein level (15 g per serving). This granola also has 11 g of fiber (almost half of your day's recommended amount) per serving.

Make the whole amount and store it for everyday use. Talk about an isoflavone feast! Enjoy in moderation—1 serving (without milk or yogurt) has 372 calories and 65 g of carbohydrates.

> 1 cup honey
>
> 1 tablespoon flaxseed oil
>
> 1½ teaspoons vanilla extract

Continued

6 cups old-fashioned rolled oats

1 cup soy nuts

1 cup wheat germ

1 cup oat bran

3 cups mixed dried fruits, such as figs, pitted dates, raisins, cranberries, blueberries, apples, or apricots

Nonfat milk or yogurt for serving

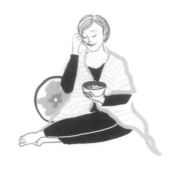

Preheat the oven to 350°F. Line 2 rimmed baking sheets (jelly-roll pans) with parchment paper.

In a large bowl, stir the honey, oil, and vanilla together. Stir in the rolled oats, soy nuts, wheat germ, and oat bran. Spread the mixture onto the prepared pans and bake for 20 minutes, or until golden brown. Remove from the oven and let cool completely. Mix in the dried fruits. Serve with milk or yogurt.

Store extra granola in an airtight covered container in the refrigerator for up to 2 weeks.

STRENGTHEN YOUR BONES WITH VITAMIN D

Glorious sunshine! It provides 90 percent of our required vitamin D through a chemical reaction in the skin. This ability decreases as we age. Sunscreen, protective clothing, and time spent indoors may also be preventing us from getting enough vitamin D, which comes from the sun's ultraviolet B rays. Vitamin D helps the body absorb calcium and phosphorous, and is found in certain foods, like fatty fish and fortified milk and juice—although we get very little from food. Supplements are one of the best ways for adults to get more of it. Before age fifty, we need at least 400 international units a day; after fifty, about 800 international units each day. Ask your doctor to test your vitamin D level.

Calcium Friendly Advice: Skip the Soft Drinks

Studies have linked soft drinks to osteoporosis, obesity, tooth decay, and heart disease. The phosphoric acid in soft drinks interferes with the body's ability to use calcium, which can lead to osteoporosis or softening of the teeth and bones. Phosphoric acid also neutralizes the hydrochloric acid in your stomach, which can interfere with digestion, making it difficult to utilize nutrients. One soda a day increases diabetes risk by 85 percent and increases obesity risk by 60 percent. This is no surprise when you consider that one can of soda has about 10 teaspoons of sugar, 150 calories, 30 to 55 mg of caffeine, and is loaded with artificial food coloring and sulphites. This is an alarming amount of sugar, calories, and harmful additives in a product that has absolutely no nutritional value. Sugar is highly addictive and creates a cascading river of health problems. Wean yourself off this stuff. Even if you drink "diet" soft drinks, you are still ingesting all the same toxic additives, and now you're adding another toxic ingredient to the mix: artificial sweetener. Drink purified or filtered water, mineral water with a slice of citrus fruit, or 100 percent unsweetened juice (whole fruits and veggies are even better!) and teas instead. Think natural and organic, always the best mantra.

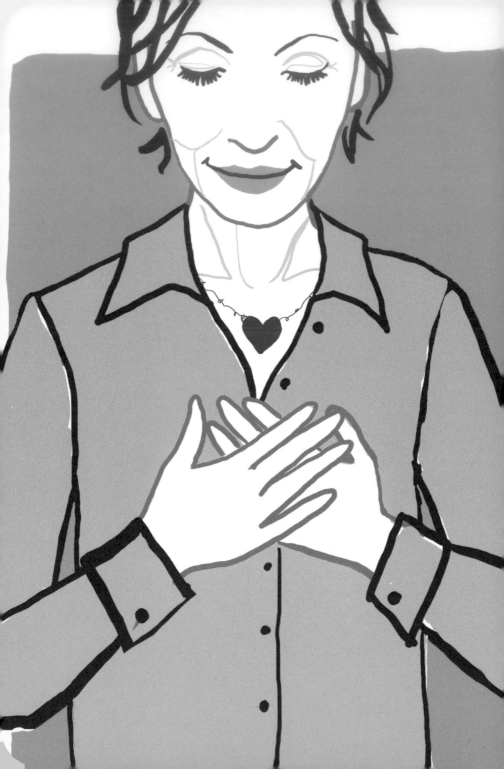

chapter 11

THE HEART OF THE MATTER

Heart disease is prevalent in our culture and on the rise within the female population. There must be a shift in how we treat our heart. It might help if we see the heart as an energetic center where we manifest compassion and love. Western medicine has typically seen the heart as a pump that transports oxygenated blood to the brain and organs. Our heart sends up to 25 quarts of blood through 60,000 miles of blood vessels every minute, and helps in circulating more than 100 million gallons in a lifetime! Each heartbeat creates an electromagnetic wave that washes over the 60 trillion cells in our body, with every one of these cells being vibrated by our heart. The heartbeat's electromagnetic frequencies can be measured up to four feet from the body. This may explain the good energy that seems to flow from some people, as well as the bad energy that others seem to project. The kind of energy that our heart manifests affects not only those around us, but is an important factor in our health. Studies show that heart patients who feel positive are 20 percent more likely to be alive a decade later than those who are morose.

OPENING THE HEART

Medical researchers have explored the heart's ability to metabolize harmony, peace, and love. Studies show that we possess incredible healing capabilities when we learn to open our heart. At the Institute of HeartMath, in Boulder Creek, California, researchers had people focus on feelings of love and appreciation whenever they began to feel emotionally overwrought: angry, frustrated, anxious, depressed. After one month the participants' levels of DHEA, an anti-aging hormone, had increased 100 percent. Levels of cortisol, a stress hormone, decreased by 23 percent. It was also found that 80 percent of study participants experienced slowed breathing rates, and that their hearts became synchronized with their breathing. In a control group, there were no physical or hormonal changes. The researchers concluded: "There are a lot of implications for health. With feelings of love the inner systems synchronize. That affects your cardiovascular system, immune system, your hormones, and even cognitive performance."

HeartMath is but one of several progressive organizations that are at the forefront of creating a new model for heart health. They provide a wide variety of tools by which we may heal, nurture, and open our heart. An integral part of this is letting our heart speak to others' hearts.

This is just one of the many techniques that can harmonize, balance, and heal the cardiovascular system, and in turn our body and mind.

+ When you feel stressful emotions, close your eyes and go inside yourself. Direct your attention to your heart, and conjure a feeling of gratitude and loving-kindness for yourself, another person, or an experience.

+ Sustain these feelings and continue to send this positive energy outward. Take deep cleansing breaths and bathe in your heart vibrations, which are sending out love and warmth. Your heart, your body, and your mind will begin to release and let go of held tension. You'll feel a tremendous sense of well-being.

+ Use whenever you feel it's appropriate. You'll know.

HEART HEALTH

Heart disease is now the leading killer of American women. Each year, 267,000 women die of heart attacks, more than six times the number of those who die from breast cancer. What to do? Consider the following:

+ Schedule a physical to check for risk factors, such as high blood pressure, high cholesterol, BMI (a measure of body fat), and blood sugar levels (a precursor to diabetes). If there is a family history of heart disease, test for risk factors like elevated homocysteine and elevated high-sensitivity C-reactive protein levels (which can indicate a 20 percent higher risk of heart disease). In women, high homocysteine levels can triple the risk of dying from heart disease. This amino acid damages artery walls, weakening them. Folic acid and B_{12} are integral in lowering homocysteine levels. Folic acid can cut homocysteine levels by as much as 25 percent!

✦ Many drugs can potentially damage a woman's heart, including antibiotics, contraceptives, diuretics, laxatives, synthetic estrogens, and even some heart drugs. These can drain our body of the nutrients that protect the heart. Magnesium is one of these nutrients. It raises HDL ("good") cholesterol, inhibits blood clotting, improves heart-muscle function, lowers blood pressure, and dilates the blood vessels. Make sure that you get at least 400 mg of magnesium a day from your diet and/or supplementation. Many fine calcium/magnesium combinations exist.

✦ Get moving. Studies show that exercise leads to a 30 to 50 percent reduction in cardiovascular disease in women. It strengthens our most important organs—the heart and lungs—and helps prevent serious problems like heart disease and diabetes. It helps us lose or stabilize weight, lowers blood pressure and cholesterol, and is great for overall heart health. Thirty minutes of walking three times a week can reduce the risk of heart attack, and walking ten or more blocks a day lowers the risk of heart disease risk by 35 percent. Studies show that an unfit person has a risk of heart attack or stroke that is eight times greater than someone who is physically fit.

✦ Control stress. It's associated with high blood pressure and an elevated heart rate. Stress hormones damage arteries, making them susceptible to plaque buildup. This applies to any suppressed or runaway emotions. Heart attacks *can* start in the mind. Those who score high on tests for anger, hostility, or depression have higher blood levels of the inflammatory markers called C-reactive proteins, which are strongly related to cardiovascular risk. Stress hormones disrupt the way that heart cells take up calcium, which is essential for heart-muscle cells to contract. (Make sure you're practicing some of the stress management therapies found in Part One of this book.)

+ Stay positive. Studies of postmenopausal women show that the most optimistic ones had very little thickening of the carotid arteries. Deal with depression as needed. Studies have shown that people rated as the most depressed had the highest levels of TNF-alpha, an inflammatory protein known to hasten heart failure.

+ Eat heart healthy: a diet low in saturated and trans fats, refined carbohydrates, and sugars, and high in whole grains, leafy greens, and "good" fats. (Good fats include the omega-3 fatty acids found in fatty fish, flax and hemp seed, and certain nuts like walnuts.) In studies, fish oil was shown to reduce heart deaths by 32 percent! It reduces inflammation and triglycerides, stabilizes heart rhythms, normalizes vascular function, and thwarts clots. (If on blood thinners, talk to your physician). Soluble fiber—the kind found in oats, barley and beans— lowers LDL and total cholesterol. And get your flavonoids, those powerful antioxidants found in fruits and vegetables (the more varied the colors of these you eat the better), along with tea and wine. They can prevent damage to blood vessel walls and help maintain the lipoproteins that carry cholesterol through the blood in their less damaging form (HDL).

+ If you smoke, quit. Smoking causes almost as many heart disease deaths as lung cancer deaths. Even five cigarettes a day can triple a women's risk for cardiovascular disease.

+ Ultimately, our task as women is to look at our lives and figure out where we fit into the world, and to understand how to deal with our negative emotions. Depression, stress, hostility, grief, and social isolation all impact our cardiac health. It has been proven that people who have no emotional support are poorest in heart health. We simply must learn to reach out and connect with others in order to heal ourselves physically and spiritually. Now surround yourself with some fragrant lavender essential oil, breathe deeply, and contemplate this goal.

Green tea is bursting with antioxidants called catechins, which have proven protective benefits against heart disease. It's also well known for its metabolism-boosting benefits, which can help burn more fat and thus control weight. And now, studies are showing that green tea significantly decreases the risk of breast cancer in post-menopausal women. Why? It "turns down" the level of circulating estrogen, which has been implicated in the development of breast cancer. Research suggests that a daily cup of green tea (bagged or loose—and organic, please!) will provide these benefits. You may derive the same benefits from a wide variety of foods, from green tea chicken noodle soup to green tea pound cake to green tea sorbet. The American Institute for Cancer Research is an excellent resource for recipes of this type. And in a pinch, there is always a green tea supplement. You may also try the following:

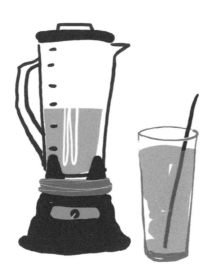

Matcha Green Tea Smoothie

Matcha green tea is made from shade-grown gyokuro leaves, whereas regular green tea is made from sencha leaves. Matcha is the green tea used in traditional Japanese tea ceremonies. This premium powder can be purchased at natural foods stores, Japanese markets, or on the Internet.

½ teaspoon matcha green tea powder

¼ cup hot water (not boiling)

1 tablespoon organic sugar or natural sweeteners to taste,
  like Stevia, agave syrup, or honey

½ cup soy milk, rice milk, or nonfat milk

1 teaspoon vanilla syrup (optional)

½ cup ice

In a bowl, combine the green tea powder and water. Whisk until completely dissolved. Stir in the sweetening and milk. Add the vanilla syrup, if you like. Place the mixture in a blender, add the ice, and blend till smooth. Enjoy!

Variation: To make a Matcha Green Tea Iced Latte, pour the mixture over ice instead of blending.

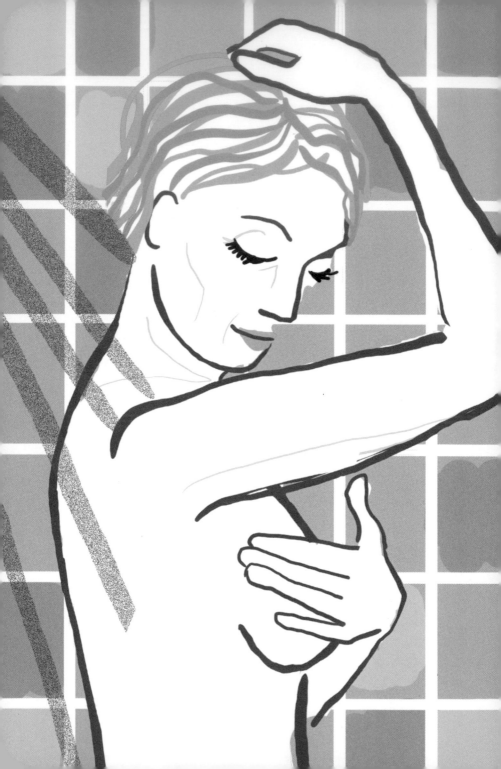

chapter 12

BREAST HEALTH

B reast health requires vigilance in self-care, life-style choices, and medical exams. The American Cancer Society now says that women today have a one-in-seven chance of developing breast cancer. Is there any wonder that so many women see this disease as a dark cloud hanging over them? Each year more than 200,000 women are diagnosed with breast cancer, and forty thousand of them will die. ❡ It is important to note that treatment for breast cancer is moving rapidly forward. Doctors now say that breast cancer must be understood as an umbrella of diseases that have different causes, arise from different types of cells, are driven by different genes, and tend to be different in women before or after menopause. For example, three-fourths of post-menopausal women have ER-positive tumors, which are those fueled by estrogen. These tumors feed off estrogen and toxins in the environment that masquerade as female hormones. Drugs like tamoxifen and a newer class of medications called aromatase inhibitors work against those cancers—whether they have spread to the lymph nodes or not.

On the other hand, women before menopause often have tumors that are ER-negative and orchestrated by bad genes. Hormone-blocking drugs may not help in these cases, and these women could benefit most from chemotherapy. This one example shows how complex and important it is that you discuss breast health with your doctor. And if you develop breast cancer, you should combine the most progressive medical practices you can find with all the mind-body healing therapies available to you.

LIFESTYLE CHOICES AND BREAST CANCER

Two lifestyle choices/factors have a tremendous impact on breast cancer: hormone replacement therapy and obesity. HRT (combining estrogen and progestin) has been found to increase the risk of first and recurrent breast cancer by 26 percent. Obesity causes the fat cells to pump out chemicals that lead to higher estrogen levels, which can generate estrogen-responsive breast tumors after menopause. Body fat also stores many environmental toxins. The less fat, the fewer toxins stored. We simply must detoxify our body of excess estrogen and poisonous toxins. Our lifestyle choices can have an impact on whether estrogen breaks down into cancer-causing or cancer-blocking compounds. Here are some choices to maintain breast health.

✦ Keep your liver as healthy as possible; it helps your body shed excess estrogen. Detox your liver through a two-pronged approach. First, reduce or eliminate your exposure to as many toxins as possible. Secondly, increase your body's ability to flush out toxins through the circulation and eliminative pathways by a variety of methods: aerobic exercise, saunas or steam baths, massages, deep healing breath, high-fiber foods, natural laxatives like psyllium, and plenty of purified or filtered water. The liver is the nucleus of our body's cleansing system, endlessly working to filter and purify our blood of toxins, with a hearty assist from the lungs, skin, kidneys, and gastrointestinal tract. The higher our exposure to toxins, the more compromised our liver function.

The many liver-fortifying foods include garlic, onions, broccoli, and artichokes. The catechins in green tea also assist liver function, as do certain minerals and antioxidants like folate. Holistic health-care providers will also prescribe a course of treatment with any one of the following herbs (preferably organic) for their liver-supportive roles: milk thistle (my personal favorite; it goes with me everywhere), licorice, dandelion, shisandra, and burdock. Confer with your primary-care physician before beginning any herbal therapy, especially if taking prescription drugs.

✦ Lessen your exposure to pesticides, hormones, and carcinogenic ingredients by buying only organic foods and natural personal-care and household cleaning products. Reduce your intake of high-fat foods (which can increase estrogen levels), particularly animal proteins. You'll reduce your exposure to carcinogens if you avoid the consumption of meat that's preserved, salted, or smoked, and also meat that's fried, broiled, or grilled at very high temperatures. Eat vegetables in abudance, especially the crucifers—broccoli, cauliflower, Brussels sprouts, cabbage—which help turn the estrogen naturally produced in your body into a cancer preventative.

✦ Give yourself regular monthly self-exams, along with a yearly medical breast exam and mammograms as guided by your doctor. Thermograms, which are more sensitive than mammograms, are also gaining in popularity.

✦ Stick to your ideal weight. Studies show that women who gain 21 to 30 pounds after age eighteen increase their risk of post-menopausal breast cancer by 40 percent. Women who gain more than 70 pounds double their risk compared with women who gained no more than 5 pounds or maintained a stable weight. (Obesity also increases the risk for a wide variety of other cancers, including endometrial, uterine, and colon.)

+ Studies have shown that moderate exercise significantly reduces serum estrogens. Three and one-half hours a week of sweat-producing exercise can cut your chances of breast cancer in half. Research studies show that the more exercise you do over your lifetime, the greater the reduction in breast-cancer risk.

+ One glass of an alcoholic beverage per day raises risk by 9 percent—and exponentially goes up from there. If you're going to drink in moderation (one a day), make certain that you're getting 400 mg of folic acid a day, which studies indicate counteracts the effects of alcohol.

+ Skip soy supplements, instead opting for the real deal. Soy has a high level of isoflavones, which are phytoestrogens that act like estrogen in the body. Eating moderate amounts of soy 3 to 4 times per week is considered to be safe, but most supplements contain phytoestrogens at levels that are far higher than in soy foods. Please note: Some studies have shown that genistein, one of the isoflavones in soy, can stimulate the growth of estrogen-receptive breast cancer and interfere with the effectiveness of the anticancer drug tamoxifen. Women who have had estrogen-receptive tumors or are taking tamoxifen should steer clear of soy unless their doctor gives them the go-ahead.

+ Make sure you get as much of your vitamins and minerals as you can from your diet, but do consider supplementing with selenium—a common trace mineral and powerful antioxidant that studies show may help shield your breasts from cancer. We used to get ample selenium from our food, but it has greatly diminished in our food supply today —especially in large-scale industrial food production. Cilantro is loaded with it; parsley has some as well.

DID YOU KNOW?

The National Institutes of Health have said that being a night owl can raise your breast cancer risk. That's because artificial light reduces your body's production of melatonin, a hormone that suppresses tumor development. A television left on all night in your bedroom, sitting at a computer into the wee hours, or too much light seeping into the bedroom during the night can trip this reaction. And if you get up during the night to use the bathroom, use a night-light to navigate your way, rather than turning on bright lights.

MASSAGE YOUR BREASTS

Breast massage is a therapeutic modality performed on the breasts of pregnant and nursing mothers; on women who have had breast reduction or augmentation; and on women who have endured mastectomy or breast cancer treatment. But breast massage is also important for women in general. In fact, every single one of us should be massaging our breast tissue daily. Regular, gentle breast massage can lessen the risk of breast cancer, though of course it does not take the place of breast self-exams, annual medical breast exams, and mammograms as recommended by your doctor, nor is it a treatment for existing breast cancer.

Breast massage allows you to become thoroughly acquainted with your breast tissue. You'll feel comfort in knowing that you're familiar with every square inch of your breasts, and more apt to detect any changes that may occur. In some circles, breast massage is seen as a potential preventative against breast cancer, as it stimulates the flow of blood and lymph fluid through the breast tissue, removing built-up toxins.

You can massage your breasts while applying moisturizing lotion or oil to your entire body after bathing. You can also perform breast massage after having soaped up in the shower, or while languishing in the tub.

✦ Become centered and present. Breathe deeply and give loving attention to your breasts during this massage ritual.

✦ Gentle-to-moderate kneading, rubbing, and squeezing strokes with the hands are sufficient to increase lymph and blood flow through the breast. The breast can be kneaded and squeezed by cupping the palm and fingers of the hand with thumb extended outward (like a handshake). Be as intuitive and fluid as possible. After all, this should also feel good. The pads of the fingertips compressing into the breast tissue will be a more exploratory movement, as in a breast self-exam.

✦ To drain lymph fluid from the breast, use your fingers to slowly and gently smooth away from the nipple to the outer edge of the breast. Work in a radial pattern pivoting around the breast (like following spokes in a wheel from the center to the edge). Use no more pressure than what you would apply to your eyelid. Too much pressure can flatten the lymphatic vessels and stop the flow of fluids and toxins.

✦ Gently massage the breast with a kneading motion, using lifting and pressing movements.

+ Slowly and carefully use your hands to twist the breast in alternating directions, being careful not to put too much tension on the breast.

+ Use both hands to apply several moderate-pressure compressions to remove more fluid.

Note: Although this is not a replacement for a monthly self-exam, if any lumps or irregularities are felt during the self-massage, confer with your doctor. Do not massage over lumps or growths until having consulted with your doctor.

FOOD FOR THOUGHT

An organic whole-foods diet can go a long way in your breast cancer prevention efforts. Beans and lentils are especially helpful, according to a recent study. Women who ate ½ cup of legumes twice a week were 24 percent less likely to develop breast cancer than women who consumed them less than once a month. The protection may come from a type of flavanol in beans and lentils.

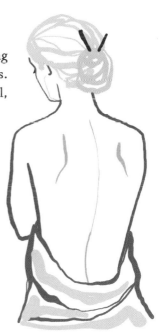

Warm Lentil Salad

The rich, smoky flavor of miso blends nicely with the earthiness of lentils in this delicious salad. Look for the green lentils and red miso at natural food stores.

1 cup green French Le Puy lentils

2 garlic cloves, minced

2 small red onions, 1 halved and 1 finely chopped

2 small carrots, peeled, 1 cut into 4 chunks and the other finely chopped

2½ cups water

½ cup finely chopped celery

1 tablespoon minced shallot

1½ tablespoons red miso

1 tablespoon red wine vinegar

1 tablespoon extra-virgin olive oil

Salt and freshly ground black pepper

In a small saucepan, combine the lentils, garlic, onion halves, carrot chunks, and water. Bring to a boil over high heat, then reduce the heat to a simmer, cover, and cook until the lentils are almost cooked through, about 15 minutes. Discard the onion and carrot chunks and add the chopped onion and carrot; continue cooking till the lentils are tender but firm, another 5 to 10 minutes.

Drain the lentils, reserving 1 tablespoon of their liquid. Pour the lentils into a medium bowl and let cool slightly. Stir in the celery and shallot.

In small bowl, cream the miso with the reserved lentil cooking liquid and the vinegar. Stir in the oil. Pour over the lentils and toss to coat. Season to taste with salt and pepper. Serve warm or at room temperature.

CONCLUSION

It's been my pleasure to serve as your menopausal muse through these pages. The healing therapies and "secrets" found here by no means constitute all the practices in the universe of menopausal self-care, but it's a pretty complete package. (And certainly, there is a plethora of available information out there through books, Web sites, associations, clubs, and seminars.) May it serve you well as you travel this new path in your life—from perimenopause through to your post-menopausal years. ❧ Women on average will have thirty more years of life once past menopause. With the most affirming lifestyle choices possible—stress management, nutrition, physical activity, connectedness to others, and a positive attitude (with a capital A!), these can be the best years of our lives. In cultures world-wide, the elder woman's wisdom, strength, optimism, and acceptance are legendary. Become a legend in your own time. Anthropologist Margaret Mead said, "There is no greater power than the zest of a postmenopausal woman." May your life be filled with zest!

INDEX

AUTHOR'S NOTE ON MEDICAL CARE

WHEN TO CALL YOUR DOCTOR

+ If you experience long-term heavy bleeding, or any bleeding one year after your period stops. This could be a sign of uterine cancer.

+ If you have any symptoms or pain that will not resolve quickly and that disrupt your sleep, work, or daily activities.

+ If you experience a drastic change in your body, such as rapid weight gain or loss, lumps or growths, extreme hair loss, abdominal bloating, and so on.

With any of the above, this is not a time to be stoic. See your doctor, and hopefully receive peace of mind that treatment and resolution of the problem are possible. And please do revisit the practices outlined in Part One of this book. Any mind-body healing approach that helps you to center yourself and deflect stress will be helpful in boosting your overall health.

DISCLAIMER

The author has done her best in preparing this book, but makes no representations or warranties with respect to the accuracy or completeness of the contents. The author and publisher disclaim any liability from any injury that may result from the use, proper or improper, of the information contained in this book. The accuracy and completeness of the information provided herein and the opinions stated herein are not guaranteed or warranted to produce any particular results, and the advice and strategies contained herein may not be suitable for every individual. The information is not intended to substitute for the knowledge and advice of your own health-care provider and your own common sense. Whenever you have concerns or questions about your health or the health of others, consult your doctor or other health-care professional. Always consult with your physician before using any of the suggestions outlined in this guidebook.

ACKNOWLEDGMENTS

My heartfelt gratitude to my editor Lisa Campbell. You are brilliant! I also want to thank everyone at Chronicle Books for your support on this project, and for giving the book such a beautiful look and feel.

I'm grateful to Dr. Toni Bark for reading through the book for medical accuracy. Your devotion to integrative medicine is so appreciated.

To the many wise women in my life—family and friends—who have truly inspired me, especially: Bea Sochor, Vi Nelson, Susan Macleary, Leslie Pace, Marsha Engle, Mary Atherton, Judy Rambert, Christie Phillips, Kathleen Bucci Bergeron, and Ann Mincey.

To my core group of beautiful yogini students (friends): Mary Lou, Nancy, Linda, Judith, Carol, and Ana.

To my mentors in the realm of women's and mind-body health—for whom wholeness in mind, body, spirit, and environment are a part of every breath you take: Dr. Christiane Northrup, Dr. Deepak Chopra, Dr. David Simon, Dr. Andrew Weil, Dr. Candace Pert, Dr. Susan Lark, Susan Weed, Althea Northage-Orr, Horst Rechelbacher, and Rod Stryker.

And to all my fellow seekers, who find the sacredness in nature, and are looking to infuse your lives with peace, creativity, joy, and love.

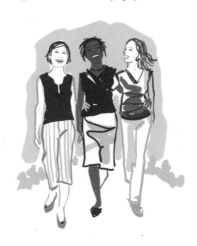